PRAISE FOR THE MENOPAUSE SWITCH

Dr. Carissa shares her professional expertise and personal experiences in an easy to understand dialog. She provides thoughtful answers and advice for every problem women face in menopause. - **Virginia A. Ward, MD**

In my opinion, every woman should read this book. Dr. Carissa Alinat expertly explains hormones and their effects on sleep, weight gain, brain fog, and sex drive in this easy-to-read book. A must for any woman who wants to have a better understanding of how their hormones affect so many aspects of their lives and how they feel. Dr. Carissa gives actionable advice on what you can do RIGHT NOW to improve your health. - **Katie Kaffai, Founder Living Young Center for Health & Anti-Aging**

Dr. Alinat is captivating and heroic in her genuine discussion on the taboo topic of 'being hormonal' and illuminates the biological underpinnings of what it is to be a woman, inspiring self-acceptance and radical insights to feeling whole again during the menopause journey. - **Lauren Wright MSN, AGNP-BC, Founder and CEO of The Natural Nipple, Microbiome + Immunity Researcher**

This book should help a lot of women and maybe even some men who have no idea about how to handle midlife. It is a good read and I like the way Dr. Carissa wrote as if sitting down to chat over a glass of resveratrol. - **Laura Boyd, P**

High praise for *The Menopaus*   D1260609   ad, but don't be fooled. It's full of 'ne   ssfully navigate menopause (before, during and after!). Finally, a down-to-earth guide with actionable steps that will help women understand what's happening and what to do to take back control of our own bodies. Thank you for empowering women with this valuable knowledge. - **Shawna Kaminski BKin, BEd, Female Health Expert & Best-Selling Author of Lose Your Menopause Belly**

Dr. Carissa has written a book that is well-researched, covering topics that are current: Unhealthy plastics and the infamous endocrine disruptors. The book is not only a pleasure to read but covers lots of excellent information put together to improve women's health and more importantly, address the adjunct therapies for going through menopause. I highly recommend it for any woman at any stage of life. **- Linda Lewallen, MD**

Before I begin, it is important to understand my relationship with Dr. Carissa Alinat, as I have known her as an incredible nurturer of children for many, many years. As a pediatrician, my relationship with mothers and women in general is crucial. I have been fortunate to help take care of thousands of first- and second-generation families in my practice for the past 30 years and my thirst for knowledge about the health of women and how it relates to their raising of children has always been of great interest to me. I have found Dr. Alinat's book to help quench that thirst as it yields fascinating insight into the changing body, mind, and soul of women as they experience and pass through menopause. The information gathered here in my journey of reading her wonderful piece of work will be invaluable as I continue my career taking care of families, especially women as mothers and grandmothers. I want to thank Dr. Carissa Alinat because I know the information her book will help me be a better pediatrician... and husband. **- Greg H. Savel, MD, FAAP, Myrtle Avenue Pediatrics, Morsani College of Medicine, University of South Florida**

As a woman in her thirties and mom of a little girl,
The Menopause Switch spoke to me in so many ways. Dr. Carissa breaks down the science of female hormones in a way that is easy to digest and puts into perspective the importance of being mindful and considerate about how everything from the products we use, birth control, exercise, and nutrition affect our hormone balance. It was empowering to read how much control I really have over what I used to think was just part of being a woman. A must-read! - **Dr. Katie Harney, Certified Nutrition Consultant, Female Fat Loss Specialist, Empowered**

THE MENOPAUSE SWITCH

Dr. Carissa Alinat is an Advanced Practice Registered Nurse (APRN) and a Doctor of Philosophy (PhD) in Nursing Science. The information found in *The Menopause Switch* is intended for educational purposes and is not intended as medical advice. You should consult your physician or other medical provider before starting this or any other weight loss, hormone therapy, exercise, or supplement program. The author and its publisher disclaim responsibility for any adverse effects resulting from this information.

The Food and Drug Administration has not evaluated the statements contained in *The Menopause Switch.*

THE
MENOPAUSE
SWITCH

Disrupt Aging & Live Your Best Life Past Midlife

By
Carissa Alinat, PhD, APRN

Foreword By
Marcelle Pick, OBGYN NP

CONTENTS

Appendices

Acknowledgments

First and foremost, I would like to acknowledge the magnificent tribe of women I have the honor of sharing my hormonal enlightenment with. To my local patients of whom I see on a regular basis as well as my readers who live afar, you make my job feel fulfilling. When I am 80, I want to look back knowing I made a mark on the world in a meaningful way. Thank you for helping me get there.

Thank you to the myriad of inspirational leaders in natural hormone balancing including Marcelle Pick. Listening to her presentation at an Institute of Functional Medicine conference sent me on a mission to help educate women worldwide on how to regain their bodies, health, and sanity. My construction of the happy hormone online railroad began that day. I am also honored that she wrote the foreword to this book.

I also owe thanks to Dr. Tami Horner and Angela Zarzycki for being there any time I need them even if it's just for a little reassurance.

A special shout out and thanks to Dr. Christine Laramée, Lauren Wright, Dr. Virginia A. Ward, Dr. Linda Lewallen, Dr. Maria-Carmen Wilson, Dr. Dan Ritchie, Laura Boyd, Dr. Katie Harney, Fritzie Abaquita, James Lloyd Clavel, Dr. Greg Savel, Shawna Kaminski, as well as Dr. Kareem Samhouri.

I am grateful for our team at Living Young Center. Katie Kaffai provided me with an amazing opportunity years ago and it has been smooth sailing since, which is rare when two hormonal women work together for so long. Sandy Kisslinger, my office manager and awesome friend, also allowed me to hide in one of our treatment rooms on lunch break so I could write.

To our "Brady Bunch," Julian, Brooke, Bradley, Brune, and Scarlett. Thank you for continuing to flourish and not resent me for the numerous times I couldn't make it to soccer games or dance practice because I had to work late or was locked in the office with my nose in research. You continue to amaze me with your perseverance at blooming into such balanced, happy, responsible, and loving little humans. I couldn't be more proud of you.

To the strongest and most selfless woman I know, my grandmother, Bea Kennedy. You have helped me in countless ways and I cherish you. To my late grandfather, Gil Kennedy, I miss you terribly. You always made such a big deal over my accomplishments and it pushed me to want to go further.

I really want to thank my chef husband, Guillaume, for he was the one who had to put up with me as I ran a busy clinic while writing this book. He loves me, he feeds me, he calms me down, and he is also the best dad ever for our agglomeration of children. I couldn't ask for a better life partner and best friend. You truly treat me like a queen.

Foreword

After practicing women's health for over 33 years, I have found that many women have problems with their hormones, be it irregular periods, premenstrual syndrome (PMS), premenstrual dysphoric disorder (PMDD), perimenopausal or menopausal changes. Women want to know what to do and how to get their hormones balanced. I've been working with many of those women over the years, looking at some of the common reasons for hormonal dysregulation. Conventional models do not consider that a lot of women have an abundance of hormonal problems which leaves many with unanswered questions.

What should they do?

That is where *The Menopause Switch* comes in. This beautifully laid out book will help you understand what might be going on for you as an individual, and what needs to be changed.

In *The Menopause Switch*, you will read that by changing your diet, eliminating the use of a microwave and other possible toxic exposures, or by changing the amount of stress you may have in your life, you can better regulate your hormones. Many people think that hormone balancing is impossible. It's not. It is explained simply and beautifully in this book. Yes, it is possible to have a life of balance and hormonal regulation by making adjustments to your life.

Menopause can be a life-changing experience. One that makes you look in the mirror and love what you see. One that makes you feel energized, and hormonally balanced. Dr. Carissa Alinat lays out the evidence in her wonderful book.

Marcelle Pick, OBGYN and Pediatric Nurse Practitioner
Co-Founder of Women to Women Clinic
Faculty at The Institute of Functional Medicine
Author of *The Core Balance Diet, Is It Me or My Adrenals?* And *Is It Me or My Hormones?*

Introduction

After sitting in the waiting room for an hour, Sandra was escorted to a cold, sterile room by a medical assistant who spent a few minutes reviewing her medication list and allergies before her doctor came in. Sandra, according to her file, was fifty-two years old and taking blood pressure and cholesterol medications, along with an antidepressant. "How can I help you today?" Sandra broke out into a sweat. "I can't sleep at night. I fall asleep fine but I wake up drenched and then I have a hard time falling back asleep. Is there something that can be done about this?" The doctor clicked his computer mouse several times. "It's most likely menopause, this is normal. Don't worry, it won't last forever. But I'll send a prescription for some sleeping pills that should help." In seven minutes, which is the average time a doctor spends with a patient, Sandra had asked for help to relieve her symptoms but instead of addressing the root cause of her sleep issues, which were night sweats caused by menopause, her doctor put her on another medication that would simply mask the problem.

Not everyone shares the same story as Sandra but if you're reading this book, you are most likely part of the 75% of women who seek help for menopause symptoms and don't receive it. Maybe you are struggling with hot flashes, night sweats, and sleeplessness. Maybe you just don't feel like you used to and want to find that happy inner diva again. Or maybe you are more concerned with your looks: Your hair is not growing where you want it to but popping up where you don't.

Regardless of how you physically feel, the onset of menopause means a marked increase in certain health risks. For example, hormonal changes can result in an accelerated rise in LDL "bad" cholesterol in the year following menopause, boosting the possibility of heart disease. And though both men and women often suffer a loss of bone density with age, the sudden reduction in estrogen associated with menopause has been shown to trigger an inflammatory reaction in some women that leads to a dramatic decrease in bone mass. Let's face it: Women experience osteoporosis twice as much as men do.

I'm here to help. What if I told you that everything you have been taught about menopause, that it's an inevitable decline in women's health and wellbeing and there's nothing you can do about it, is a lie? What if I told you reinvention is possible at any age and you can achieve the highest possible level of wellness after the first half of your life?

The word "menopause" stems from Latin words meaning "monthly stop," referring to the cessation of your menstrual cycle. It does not mean your life stops. In fact, for many women, this is just the start of a beautiful new beginning. It's time to switch from a negative mindset of giving up to a brand new positive attitude that there's a bump in the road and it's time to mend it so you can cruise through the rest of your life feeling vibrant, healthy, happy, and confident. You can live intentionally again. You can be victorious. There's a quote by Carl Jung that I adore:

"Life really does begin at forty.
Up until then, you are just doing research."

Midlife presents an opportunity to take the wisdom that you have gained, the knowledge you have attained, and the courage you have acquired to live out your best life with confidence, freedom, and an "it's about me now" attitude.

This is not snake oil. My education, experience in clinical research trials, ability to pick apart peer-reviewed randomized clinical trials, and my hands-on experience with patients at my clinic, has helped me create this step-by-step guide to helping women find balance naturally and effectively. With that being said, I am also careful not to overdeliver. Sometimes eating, exercising, detoxing, and supplementation just isn't enough. That means I do prescribe bioidentical hormones when I deem it necessary, but I often offer natural, effective treatments to try first.

I'm a nurse practitioner with a PhD in research. I run a busy clinic in Florida and I treat women's hormones through a functional medicine approach. I also have experience working on multimillion-dollar clinical trials. This means I can dig through piles upon piles of research studies to find the best scientific evidence. I'm a wife. I understand that balanced hormones are essential for keeping a sane marriage or relationship. I'm a mother. I understand that balanced hormones are also essential for keeping a sane family life. I'm a daughter. I know that hormone imbalances often run in families and cause harm. Obesity, depression/anxiety, fibrocystic breasts, and uterine fibroids run in my family. Both my mother and grandmother had hysterectomies in their 20's. I'm a woman. Just like you, I have been confused about what's happening within my body and looked for answers. The answers weren't in the most obvious places but through years of research, education, and blood, sweat, and tears, *The Menopause Switch* was developed, tested, found to be effective, and it has already helped so many women in my practice. Now, it's available to you and thousands of other women around the world, too.

The Menopause Switch is divided into three parts. *Part I: Hormones 101* equips you with the fundamentals. Chapter 1 provides a basic primer on what hormones are, with focus on the top 3 that are most likely to cause you to feel crummy during midlife. Chapters 2 and 3 describe the different stages in a woman's reproductive life, the hormonal shifts that occur starting from the first time a woman gets her period until years after it ends, what problems can go awry, affecting the way she feels, especially around the time of menopause.

Part II: Preparing for the Menopause Switch educates you on what goes in our mouths, what touches our skin, what we breathe in, how we cope with stress, how our genes behave, all affect our hormones. Based on exhaustive detective work, I have created a step-by-step guide on how to lower the toxic load in your environment, in your body, and in your mind, so that you can put back into harmony your delicate balance of hormones, so you can regain your vitality.

Part III: Flipping the Menopause Switch hones in on the most common midlife complaints with targeted lifestyle changes, neutraceutical and botanical therapies to help reduce or eliminate bothersome menopausal symptoms. These recommendations are based on a robust amount of research, as you will notice from my vast amount of references.

Part IV: Recipes will take you into your own kitchen, where you'll learn that cooking while on menopause can be a lot of fun. My husband, Chef Gui Alinat, has put together 28 delicious recipes using my guidelines. Food has a specific impact on your body. Together we'll learn what foods you should enjoy, and which ones you should stay away from. I don't advocate for restrictive diets. Quite the contrary, my bi-yearly stays in France with my husband's family has turned me into a lover of great foods, and we tried to communicate that love to you. Embrace food.

Before we go any further, let me just say first that attitude always affects success. The most successful people in this world started out with a positive vision. Amelia Earheart didn't become the first female aviator to fly over the Atlantic Ocean because she thought her ability was lacking. Sara Blakely didn't invest her life in creating Spanx, deeming her the youngest self-made female billionaire in 2012, if she didn't believe in it. Okay, so maybe these examples aren't exactly at the same parallel with menopause but you get my point – people don't succeed without having a vision first. So, if hot flashes, sleeping difficulties, and weight gain are dragging you down but you don't think there's anything you can do to fix them, you don't need another book on menopause, you need a vision makeover. If you have a vision that you can reclaim your body, your sanity, and your happiness, then you've come to the right place. This book will help you live out your vision.

Be your "GOAT"; Be your Greatest of All Time.

PART ONE

Hormones 101

CHAPTER 1

HORMONE BASICS

"A woman is like a tea bag – you can't tell how strong she is until you put her in hot water." — Eleanor Roosevelt

At some point, you've probably heard someone say, "Sorry, I'm just being hormonal." When things aren't going right and you don't feel quite like yourself, you can blame it on your hormones.

Why? Because your body is ruled by hormones, so you can tell your husband that the next time he annoyingly leaves the toilet seat up and you angrily set his underwear on fire.

Women come to my clinic for a variety of reasons. Mostly, I hear about obvious symptoms such as having hot flashes so severe they contribute to global warming, but I also hear about ambiguous symptoms such as "brain fog." For some women, menopause is a smooth sail upon tranquil waters. They don't hit any bumps whatsoever; their period stops and it's just business as usual. For others, menopause is more like waterskiing across puddles of hot lava. Their periods stop for 2 months and return, then gone for 3 months and return, all meanwhile sweating in misery and wondering when it's ever going to end.

Many women I have met in the hot lava lake of menopause say this same exact sentence: "I want to try natural first." This is your guide to doing just that.

Eve Ate from the Apple and Now She Suffers

Unfortunately for us, women seem to be more vulnerable to hormonal imbalances than men. Women are prescribed thyroid medications almost ten times more than men[1], as well as antidepressants and anti-anxiety medications almost twice as much[2].

Why such a big difference? Well, for one thing, we go through more hormonal changes in our lives than men. Our monthly hormonal rollercoaster when we get periods is a good example. Another is getting pregnant, growing another human being inside of us for nine months, giving birth, and possibly breastfeeding up to a year or more. It takes a lot of hormonal fluctuations to make all that possible.

What's a Hormone Anyway?

Hormones... What are these little control freaks residing in our bodies? The existence and function of hormones is a newer discovery in the realm of modern science. In 1905, English physician E.H. Starling and physiologist W.M. Bayliss were the first to coin the word 'hormone,' which in Greek means "to arouse or excite" and told the rest of the world about their new discovery that "the chemical messengers which are speeding from cell to cell along the blood stream, may coordinate the activities and growth of different parts of the body" [3]. In short, hormones are little chemical messengers that are produced in one part of your body but have effects on other parts of your body. From simple things like how fast your heart beats when you're under stress, to more complex processes like fertility and reproduction. Hormones affect nearly every single process in our bodies. Each hormone has a job to do. For example, the adrenal glands produce a very powerful hormone called cortisol, which helps you wake up in the morning and get your day going. When something stressful happens, extra cortisol is released to help get you through it. Your ovaries produce many hormones, such as estrogen, progesterone, and testosterone, and their main jobs are to help you reproduce. Your thyroid gland produces thyroid hormones, which help keep your body temperature where it should be so you don't need to lay in the sun like a lizard to stay warm even though it's 80 degrees out.

Let's start with Hormones 101 to set the foundation for the rest of the book. Once you understand the hormone basics then you will be able to understand why it's important to make a few tweaks in your lifestyle in order to find balance and feel better.

The Balancing Act

Everything in our body, on Earth and in the Universe requires balance. We would not be alive if there was no balance of gravity between the Earth and Sun, balance among the gases in which we breathe, or among the nutrients in the soil in which we grow food. Our bodies are no different. There is a complex, delicately balanced system that needs to be in place for us to live. Our bodies need to be in constant homeostasis, or, in stable conditions, in order for us to not only survive but also feel our very best. Aging, stress, and illness can make this difficult. Our hormones play a huge role in keeping homeostasis or balance in our bodies and if hormones aren't balanced themselves, then well, "Houston, we have a problem." A homeostasis problem, that is.

Homeostasis: From the Greek words for "same" and "steady," refers to any process that living things use to actively maintain fairly stable conditions necessary for survival [4].

How does this balance occur? The process of how hormones are balanced in the body starts in the hypothalamus located in the brain, which sends signals to the nearby pituitary gland, also known as the "master gland." The pituitary gland then communicates with other glands in the body which are responsible for producing other hormones. There are a dozen glands in our body including the hypothalamus, pituitary, pineal, adrenal, thyroid, pancreas, ovaries, and more. There are feedback loops between the brain and hormones to keep levels where they should be. The body can sense when hormone levels are low or high and signals are sent out to increase or decrease the amount of hormones being produced. Think of it as a thermostat. For example, the thyroid gland is like a thermostat. If the body is too hot, the thyroid gland will send a hormone to the brain to tell it to slow down its signal back to the thyroid gland to change the temperature. Hence the temperature will adjust. In addition, hormones interact with each other and affect levels of each. For example, cortisol levels rise in the morning (helping you wake) as melatonin levels fall. In reverse, melatonin levels rise in the evening (helping you sleep) as cortisol levels fall. Everything is interrelated, like an orchestra. All the parts need to play well because if one is off, it will affect the symphony.

Birth of a Hormone

A step to understanding hormone imbalances is to become familiar with the body's natural hormonal cascade. The reason why this is important is because one hormone imbalance can lead to another. For example, severe stress can cause an imbalance in cortisol hormone. If cortisol hormone production remains high, it can cause other hormone levels to be low.

The birth of a hormone begins with cholesterol. Cholesterol is the main ingredient when it comes to making hormones in the body. The first hormone made from cholesterol is called pregnenolone, also known as the "mother hormone." This hormone "cascades" into other hormones. In fact, it separates into two chains: One chain forms progesterone, aldosterone, and cortisol, and the other forms dehydroepiandrosterone (DHEA), testosterone, and estrogen. However, abnormal circumstances such as stress can cause an interruption in the normal hormone cascade. Again, when you experience chronic stress, you make more cortisol (hence known as the stress hormone). Since your body needs more cholesterol to make more cortisol when you're highly stressed, there's less left to make other hormones like progesterone.

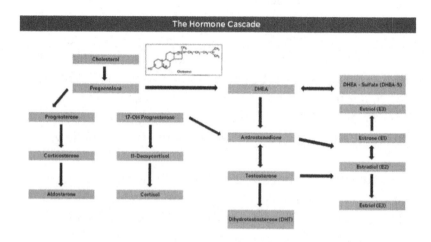

The Hormone Cascade

Hormones: Unlocking the Doors

You may be wondering, "If hormones travel throughout your body, what happens when they get to their destination?" Well, what happens when you get home from work and the door is locked? You use your key to open it. Every organ that is targeted by a hormone contains cells. Some of those cells have locks called receptors. Only the specific hormone (the key), can unlock the receptor by binding to it. Once there is a connection between the hormone and the receptor, the signal gets through and its job is done. However, sometimes the receptors don't work like they should. That's why even if a hormone level shows up as "normal" on a blood test, it might mean that you have plenty of hormone floating around in your bloodstream but you *feel* like its low because it's not getting inside of your cells to do its job. It's important to keep this in mind when it comes to menopause. Many women suffer from symptoms of low testosterone even though their levels are regarded as "within range" on a blood test.

The Holy Trinity of Hormones

There are so many different hormones that help your body function like the super complex organism it is. There are about 50 different hormones in the body and scientists may discover more [5]. When it comes to the time around menopause, there is a hormonal trinity that needs to be in balance for you (and consequently whoever else is around you so they don't suffer too) to experience true peace and happiness. All hormones are important but there are three that can put you in limbo during menopause and those include estrogen, progesterone, and testosterone, which we will focus on.

Estrogen

Like Shania Twain says, "I feel like a woman!" Estrogen is what makes women feel like women. It's what teenage girls crave as they move on from stuffing their bras with toilet paper to filling in cups on their own. It's also what we crave again as we approach menopause and our once perky breasts start to droop. It's what makes us feel sexy, spicy, and vibrant. However, estrogen can become your "frenemy" around the time of menopause. During the period of perimenopause, the stage before your period has completely stopped for good, estrogen often goes up and down, with levels too high one day and too low the next. This hormonal rollercoaster ride can leave you moody, hot flashing like a campfire, drenching your bed sheets with night sweats, and suffering from the other perils of midlife.

Estrogen is an umbrella term for a group of sex hormones that promote the development and maintenance of female characteristics of the body. Three major estrogens include estrone (E1), estradiol (E2), and estriol (E3).

- Estradiol (E2): This is the strongest form of estrogen, which the body can convert back to a weaker form called estrone.
- Estrone (E1): This is the second weakest form of estrogen that is highest in women after menopause. The body can convert this into a stronger form of estrogen called estradiol.
- Estriol (E3): This is the weakest form of estrogen and is the highest during pregnancy. It cannot be converted into other types of estrogen and is actually just a waste product after the body uses its main estrogen, estradiol.

Number 2 is, in fact, number 1 in your body -- Estradiol (E2) is the head honcho of female sex hormones. It runs the show on everything from heart health to bone growth. Meanwhile, Estriol (E3) and Estrone (E1) are its minor sidekicks. Estriol has been studied for its protective effects against breast cancer [6].

Estrogens are amazing hormones and have over 400 different functions in a woman's body. They are responsible for the difference between female and male bodies. In females, they make the bones smaller and shorter, the pelvis broader, and the shoulders narrower. This group of hormones is responsible for promoting the development and maintenance of female sexual characteristics in the human body including breasts, pubic and armpit hair, and regulation of the menstrual cycle and reproductive system. Estrogens are best known for the role they play in sexual development and reproduction, but, like any modern woman, estrogens are multitaskers that wear many important hats and also have a place in many other systems in the body including the neuroendocrine, cardiovascular, skeletal and immune systems. They also act as "house manager," contributing to the overall balance in the body.

The main estrogen factory in the female body is the ovaries. The adrenal glands also make estrogens but in smaller amounts. Adipose (fat) tissues also produce estrogen. This is why overweight and obese women tend to have more estrogen and are more likely to suffer from "Estrogen Dominance" (we will get into that later) than their leaner peers. However, no matter their size, many women will eventually suffer from the effects of low estrogen.

Common symptoms of low estrogen include:

- Hot flashes
- Night sweats
- Mood swings or depression/anxiety
- Sleep difficulties
- Difficulty concentrating/Brain fog
- Dry skin and hair
- Weight gain or increase in belly fat
- Vaginal dryness, painful intercourse
- Headaches or an increase in pre-existing migraine occurrences
- Fatigue
- Low libido
- Irregular, short, light, or absent periods
- Increase in urinary tract infections (UTIs)
- Frequent urination, leaky bladder

Although commonly thought to be "the female hormone," estrogen is found in both men and women in differing amounts. Women generally have more estrogen than men, which is why it is considered to be a female hormone, while men have more testosterone, which is why it is considered to be a male hormone. But both men and women have the same hormones in their bodies, just in differing amounts, which are constantly working to find a balance for optimal functioning. Man or woman, each body has its own ideal balance when it comes to hormones and that can change every...single....day. It's important to remember that your hormone levels are not always the same, they are constantly ebbing and flowing like the tides, constantly adapting and attempting to find the right balance as things change in your body and also around you. This is influenced by every facet of your life, from your stress levels, to your diet, to your environment, and even by your genetics.

Finally, as we age, the estrogen/testosterone ratio decreases. This means that you will see women developing male sexual characteristics such as facial hair and men often develop female sexual characteristics such as breasts. Maybe if we were to live 150 years old, men and women would be alike.

Progesterone

In women, estrogen is balanced by another hormone in the body, progesterone. Progesterone is one of the primary hormones made by the ovaries and adrenal glands in menstruating women, along with estrogen and testosterone. Progesterone is actually not a sex hormone at all, as it doesn't contribute to your female sexual characteristics. However, it plays a huge role in your reproductive life and how you feel. Progesterone, while an active hormone on its own, is also a precursor to estrogen and other hormones. That means progesterone can convert into estrogen and other hormones through the cascade.

Progesterone is the Aphrodite of hormones and peacemaker within. Progesterone spikes around the time of ovulation, and along with testosterone, puts you "in the mood for love." It protects your growing baby when you're pregnant and its decline after birth triggers your body, along with another hormone prolactin, to produce milk for your new little bundle of joy. Considered to be a "calming" hormone, it's no wonder that most women feel their best in their third trimester of pregnancy when progesterone production is very high but then suffer from postpartum depression or "baby blues" when production drops after childbirth. It's also no wonder that some women feel anxious and depressed when their body stops making progesterone around the time of menopause.

Common symptoms of low progesterone include:

- Depression/Anxiety
- Mood swings

- Fatigue
- Bloating
- Tender breasts
- Low libido
- Sleeping difficulties
- Weight gain
- Increased fat in butt and hip area
- Irregular, heavy periods
- Increased PMS
- Headaches or an increase in pre-existing migraine occurrences
- Difficulty concentrating/Brain fog
- Hot flashes

When Estrogen Becomes a Dominatrix

No, estrogen dominance is not the newest installment of 50 Shades of Grey. It is a common clinical condition that results from an imbalance between estrogen and progesterone. Estrogen dominance occurs when the equilibrium, or balance, of sex hormones is shifted to favor estrogen, resulting in too much estrogen in the body. In addition, because of the influence of progesterone on the body, estrogen dominance can also be caused by low progesterone (even in the face of normal estradiol levels). Because of all the roles estrogen plays, an imbalance in the estrogen/progesterone ratio has been linked to many acute and chronic conditions, including infertility, obesity, osteoporosis, endometriosis and certain types of cancer [7], as well as thyroid dysfunction, blood clots, and stroke [8]. It can also harm tissues and lead to autoimmune diseases.

> **Side Note:** Do you think that just because you're approaching menopause, having too much estrogen is impossible for you? Wrong. This commonly happens as menopause approaches, during the perimenopausal stage, which can last for years, causing your estrogen level to go up and down like a rollercoaster until it finally stops.

Signs & Symptoms of Estrogen Dominance

There are a range of signs and symptoms that occur when your hormones are off balance and estrogen has become the dominant hormone. Unfortunately, many of these symptoms, like bloating, swollen and tender breasts, decreased sex drive, mood swings, headaches and trouble sleeping, can often overlap with other hormone imbalances. Other symptoms could include lumpy breasts (such as in fibrocystic breast disease), increased PMS side effects, anxiety, weight gain, hair loss, fatigue and memory problems. As women, we tend to push aside things like fatigue, PMS, and mood swings and chock them up to everyday life, but these side effects can be puzzle pieces to clue your doctor in on what to test for. Be sure to take time to be mindful of your body and any changes you see in the way you feel.

Symptoms of Estrogen Dominance

- Weight gain
- Fluid Retention
- Fatigue
- Headaches/Migraines
- Depression
- Anxiety
- Irregular Menstrual Cycle
- Heavy Menstrual Cramps
- Infertility
- Brain Fog
- Fibrocystic Breasts
- Tender Breasts
- Decreased Sex Drive

What's to blame?

Because it is such a complex hormone, deeply integrated into so many systems, it is often hard to pinpoint the direct cause. Obesity is well-known to be the cause of too much estrogen in the body [9] but the inflammatory nature of daily life may also increase estrogen levels and fuel estrogen dominance.

Many of the additives found in consumer household, food and beauty products contain xenoestrogens (chemicals that act like estrogen hormone), which have been studied for their role in endocrine disruption/hormone imbalance. Another cause for estrogen dominance could stem from genetics. Additionally, estrogen dominance can also result from medications like synthetic hormone replacement therapy drugs. Further, as with most diseases, chronic stress, poor diet, excess body fat, poor gut health, smoking, alcohol abuse, and exposure to toxic chemicals can all be contributing factors.

Testosterone

Testosterone is one of the most overlooked hormones that women going through menopause need more of to feel their best. It is an "androgen" hormone we generally associate with men. If estrogen is considered feminine, then testosterone is considered the masculine hormone. However, like I mentioned before, both men and women have estrogen, progesterone and testosterone in their bodies, just in differing amounts. In women testosterone is mostly secreted by the ovaries but the adrenal glands also produce around 25%. When the sex organs (i.e. ovaries) and adrenal glands are healthy, our bodies are capable of regulating testosterone levels naturally, unless we have an underlying condition prohibiting this. Levels also fall as we age.

Testosterone is what makes us feel sexy and energetic around the time of ovulation and as you can probably guess, it's part to blame for menopausal women with low libido and energy. Testosterone also helps maintain reproductive tissue and bone mass levels. However, as you read on, you will notice levels can vary drastically among women. Let's explore why having too much or too little testosterone in the body can make women feel lousy. You'll notice that the symptoms of low testosterone overlap with symptoms of low estrogen.

Common symptoms of low testosterone in women

- Low libido
- Difficulty reaching orgasm
- Vaginal dryness
- Fatigue
- Weight gain, especially around the midsection
- Brain fog/Difficulty concentrating
- PMS symptoms (bloating, headaches, fatigue, moodiness, skin changes, heart palpitations, and shortness of breath)
- Sleep disturbances (especially night sweats)
- Loss of muscle/Muscle weakness
- Sluggishness
- Loss of bone density
- Irregular menstrual cycles

PCOS: When Testosterone Takes Over

Low testosterone isn't the only possibility in women. I have noticed a rise in the increase of Polycystic Ovarian Syndrome (PCOS), a hormonal disorder, in my clients over the years, which is associated with high levels of testosterone. PCOS is the most common reproductive disorder in the United States, affecting more than 5 million women, or an estimated 6%-10% of the population. This is a condition involving enlarged ovaries with small cysts on the outer edges. Scientists are not quite sure of the cause, yet they believe there are genetic and environmental factors at play.

Symptoms of PCOS

- Irregular menstrual cycles
- Acne
- Obesity (PCOS is only found in 10% of lean women)
- Excessive hair growth
- Depression

Risk factors for PCOS

- Insulin resistance
- Elevated triglycerides
- High blood pressure
- Low levels of HDL (the good cholesterol)
- High levels of LDL (otherwise known as the bad cholesterol)

High levels of testosterone in women can also cause:

- Increased muscle mass
- Enlarged clitoris
- Acne
- Deeper voice
- Hair thinning and balding

PCOS is linked to diabetes and as a consequence, heart disease. The risk of heart disease becomes higher when the above risk factors are present. This is a serious condition and you should always work together with your doctor to manage it as sometimes medications are necessary. Unfortunately, menopause doesn't cure PCOS and it is possible that the metabolic abnormalities in women with PCOS may also worsen with age [10]. Research on women with PCOS suggest that waist circumference, LDL cholesterol, and triglyceride levels increase in women with PCOS as they reach 40 to 50 years [11].

CHAPTER 2
PREMENOPAUSE

"Women complain about PMS, but I think of it as the only time of the month when I can be myself." — *Roseanne Barr*

I'm sure you remember it as vividly as I do — the day you got your first period. In middle school, my friends and I eagerly awaited our turn. It seemed like such a mystical entry into womanhood at the time. An official sign that I would no longer be a girl, but a woman. We were all waiting for it, but few of us knew exactly what to expect.

Premenopause is just as its name suggests — the time before menopause. This can include any time in the decades between the onset of menstruation and the onset of menopause symptoms. This time is unique to each woman. It may or may not involve regular periods, fertility, pregnancy, breastfeeding, and all that comes with a monthly cycle.

Premenopause should not be confused with perimenopause. The difference between the two lies in the presence of menopause symptoms. Over the course of your menstrual lifetime, hormones are constantly changing, but it isn't until the telltale signs of menopause appear that you are considered to move out of the premenopause phase and into the perimenopause phase. This transition usually occurs when a woman is in her 40s or 50s, but can occur earlier or later for some women. So, let's dive into what exactly is going on in our bodies from that first mystical period.

From Training Bras to Tampons

The onset of menstruation and onset of puberty are two different events in a woman's life. Puberty is marked by the growth of breast tissue and increase in height. These events are followed by the onset of menstruation, which is influenced by a myriad of factors including genetics, environment, personal attributes, and lifestyle.

Mom Jeans and Genes: You're Gonna Wear 'Em Too

Our biological time clocks are passed down through our genetic code. Yes, you are very much like your mother, even if you never wanted to be. The age at which we begin our cycle seems to be strongly influenced by our mothers' age of menstruation [12]. The same goes for the age we hit menopause. Whenever your mom went through menopause naturally (without surgical removal of her reproductive organs), you're more likely to be that age as well.

The Environment is Turning Girls into Women... Earlier

The average age a girl starts her period is roughly 12 years old in the United States, but it can occur as early as 8 years old [13]. Aunt Flo is coming earlier than before. Over the last century, the age at which girls hit puberty has significantly decreased, falling by an average of about 3 months per decade. This change is controversial: Either the improvement of overall health of the general population is due to industrialization [12] or the overexposure to toxic hormone disruptors in our food and environment [14] is increasing estrogen in our bodies, as a result of industrialization.

Puberty and Periods: Size Matters

Personal attributes play a large role in the onset of puberty and menstruation. Varying body mass index (BMI) and height are strongly correlated with the age of menstruation. Basically, the more body fat girls have, the more likely they will hit puberty at an early age. There is even data that suggests that birth weight and the rate at which a baby grows in the first few months of life can affect the age of menstruation [12].

Lifestyles of the Caloric-Rich and Fertile

Nutrition and activity also seem to play an important role. Highly caloric diets and diets high in animal protein in early childhood have been associated with an earlier start. Athletes have been shown to have a delayed onset of menstruation, indicating that intense exercise can delay both puberty and menstruation [12].

The Menstrual Cycle

While most of us are fully (and painfully) aware of the symptoms of menstruation, many of us may feel as clueless as we did in middle school about what exactly is happening during our cycle. At times, menstruation can certainly feel like an aimless, wild ride, but there is a calculated plan to the ebb and flow of a woman's hormones over her lifetime. Those special few days a month when a woman is menstruating may take the spotlight, but your body is working around the clock in an intricate series of hormonal shifts to regulate your cycle. All of this is to prepare for a possible pregnancy. Unfortunately, we can't cue our reproductive organs about our plans for pregnancy, so every month, our bodies get fully ready just in case. If only we could be that prepared in our day-to-day life!

The menstrual cycle occurs in 4 phases:

1. **Menstruation.** The thickened lining of your uterus (endometrium) sheds from the body. On average, this lasts 3-7 days.

2. **Follicular phase.** This phase begins on the first day of menstruation. First, your ovary gets ready to recruit an egg while pumping out estrogen. Follicle stimulating hormone (FSH) is released from the pituitary gland in your brain, sending a message to your ovary to produce follicles (like tiny sacs) that contain immature eggs. Usually only one follicle will mature into an egg while the others die, so consider yourself

the lucky one. This occurs around day 10 of a 28-day cycle. The growth of the follicles stimulates the lining of the uterus to thicken in preparation for a possible pregnancy.

3. **Ovulation phase.** The increase in estrogen during the follicular phase stimulates the release of luteinizing hormone (LH), which triggers the start of the ovulation phase. During this phase, the egg chosen to grow in the follicles of your ovaries is released and takes a trip down the fallopian tube with the intent of being fertilized by sperm. This egg is on a mission, completely unaware of your actual plans. This phase is when you are fertile and able to get pregnant. For most, ovulation happens on or around day 14. If sperm doesn't fertilize it within 24 hours, the egg dies. Testosterone levels spike just before ovulation, putting you "in the mood." Having sex in the days leading up to ovulation can still result in pregnancy, as sperm can live in the body, on the prowl for up to 7 days.

4. **Luteal phase.** The luteal phase wraps up the cycle. During this phase the egg goes through changes and progesterone is released, along with a smaller amount of estrogen. If fertilization occurs, your body kicks into gear and produces human chorionic gonadotropin (hCG). This is the hormone that tips off pregnancy tests. If the egg goes unfertilized, estrogen and progesterone levels begin to decrease and this triggers menstruation. Since the uterus will not be used as a home for a fertilized egg, it begins to shed its lining and your period begins, starting the cycle all over again.

During the premenopausal phase of your life, periods are happening every month because your hormone production is regular (unless you have PCOS or some other underlying condition). When you start noticing your periods are becoming less predictable, that's when premenopause is most likely ending and you're headed to the next phase in your life: perimenopause.

CHAPTER 3
PREMENOPAUSE & MENOPAUSE

"Probably the happiest period in life most frequently is in middle age, when the eager passions of youth are cooled, and the infirmities of age not yet begun; as we see that the shadows, which are at morning and evening so large, almost entirely disappear at midday." —
Eleanor Roosevelt

Being a woman is a wild ride, am I right? Just when you think you've got the hang of this whole monthly cycle thing, life throws you a curve. That curve is commonly referred to as perimenopause, or the beginning of your journey to menopause. Many people think that menopause is like a flip that is switched, but it doesn't happen overnight. The journey into menopause is a process that happens over time, commonly called perimenopause or the menopausal transition. You can think of perimenopause as an in-between phase. You're winding down the premenopause phase of your life, but you're not quite ready for menopause. It's a time of transition, where your body is getting ready to say goodbye to the reproductive phase (and monthly periods!). It's a preparation to enter a new phase of being.

While not clearly defined, professionals agree that perimenopause is a time full of profound shifts in your hormones and reproductive system. On average, a woman enters perimenopause in her late 40s or early 50s. Perimenopause lasts two to eight years preceding a woman's final period and a year after the final period [15].

Perimenopause occurs in two phases:

1. Early transition, which is when your monthly period is mostly regular with a few irregular months.

2. Late transition, when you have a space of at least 60 days between periods.

The late transition comes to an end with what will be your final menstrual period.

The Mystery of Menopause

It's still unclear what really causes menopause. However, a theory exists that a woman is born with all of her follicles (sacs in the ovaries that store immature eggs) and that over time as a woman loses some with each menstrual cycle, she becomes less fertile and her ovaries stop responding to her brain's signal to produce more hormones to keep going as an attempt to reproduce. Because the ovaries aren't responding, the brain keeps surging out a signal to them to try to get them to make more hormones, and that's when hot flashes are most likely to occur. Periods can become irregular or just stop altogether. Postmenopause is defined as when a woman has not had a period for at least 12 months.

Poor nutrition and stress have traditionally been blamed for triggering early menopause. In part, that may be true. Think about it this way: Your female body was engineered to produce children. Mother Nature insists that your body be healthy enough to do that. If you don't have proper nutrition even just for yourself, you won't have proper nutrition for another human growing inside of you. Similarly, a state of constant stress is also not a good environment for a baby. Chronic stress can cause inflammation, which isn't good for a growing baby. So, if you have been dealing with stress for a long period of time, your body knows it's not an optimal time to become pregnant so it shuts down your ability to be able to do so. Regardless if you still want to be fertile or not, aiming for optimal nutrition, exercise, and stress management is ideal if you want to keep your hormones in balance in order to feel good.

Hormonal Shifts

The changes experienced in perimenopause are directly connected to hormonal shifts. Most people think that falling levels of estrogen are the main blame for why women feel so crummy during perimenopause. Here's a shocker: Menopause is not an estrogen deficiency disease. Estrogen levels only drop between 40 to 60% at menopause, while progesterone drops to nearly zero. Most women start having anovulatory cycles in their mid-30's, which means their ovaries are not releasing mature eggs even though they are still having periods. Progesterone levels drop below normal while estrogen goes unbalanced. While estrogen levels will decrease during menopause, the truth is, estrogen levels do not fall appreciably until after a woman's last period.

Perimenopause and Menopause: What's the Difference?

The difference between perimenopause and menopause is very simple. Being in menopause means that it has been at least 12 months since you had a menstrual period. When I say 12 months, I mean 12 straight months in a row. If your period is still popping up every now and then, that means your ovaries are still producing hormones and you are still in perimenopause. When your period stops completely and doesn't return, your ovaries are no longer producing enough estrogen, progesterone, or testosterone.

Menopause can happen in your forties but the average age is fifty-one in the United States. Menopause that occurs before age 40 is called early or premature menopause and can happen for a number of reasons:

- **Family history.** Women with a family history of early or premature menopause are more likely to have early or premature menopause.

- **Smoking.** Women who smoke may reach menopause as much as two years before nonsmokers and research suggests that they also die about two years earlier than non-smokers [16]. They may also suffer from more severe menopause symptoms [17].

- **Certain health conditions:** Autoimmune diseases, HIV and AIDS, genetic disorders such as Turner's syndrome, chronic fatigue syndrome.

- **Certain medications:** Chemotherapy or pelvic radiation treatments for cancer. These treatments can damage your ovaries and cause your periods to stop forever or just for a while.

- **Surgery to remove the ovaries.** Surgical removal of both ovaries, called a bilateral oophorectomy, may cause menopausal symptoms right away. Your hormone levels will drop quickly and your periods will stop after this surgery.

- **Surgery to remove the uterus.** Some women who have a hysterectomy, which removes the uterus, can keep their ovaries. If this happens, you will no longer have periods but you will probably not go through menopause right away because your ovaries will continue to make hormones. However, menopause may occur a year or two earlier than expected.

My Personal Hormone Story

One of the reasons why I became so fascinated with hormones is because I spent a lot of time trying to figure out my own. After being on birth control pills in my 20's, which by the way, turned me into a depressive and overweight nutcase, my ovaries became completely confused for years and years. I suffered from Post-Birth Control Syndrome (more about what that is later), a terrible case of estrogen dominance which led to a surgeon having to drain fluid from my fibrocystic breast, adrenal fatigue, low testosterone, and a short bout of Hashimoto's thyroiditis. Since both my mother and grandmother had hysterectomies in their early 20's back when having a hysterectomy was as common as getting a tooth pulled, I also had no idea when I could expect menopause to make its grand debut. When I had enough of being exhausted, moody, and more fog in my brain than a San Franciscan winter evening, I had to do something about it. So I did my research, found out what was going on in my body and why, and how to fix it. I felt better quickly and wanted to help others so I went back to school. From years of treating women of all ages suffering from a wide array of hormone imbalances at my clinic, I figured I could reach even more women world-wide by writing this book. Here I am.

PART TWO

Preparing for the Menopause Switch

CHAPTER 4
CLEAN YOUR MIND: PRACTICING SELF LOVE & STRESS REDUCTION

"There is a fountain of youth: it is your mind, your talents, the creativity you bring to your life and the lives of people you love. When you learn to tap this source, you will truly have defeated age." —
Sophia Loren

Hormones: What's Self Love Got to Do with It?

The purpose of this chapter is two-fold: Letting go of negative self-perceptions and taking care of yourself, combined with reducing stress that causes inflammation may contribute to optimal hormone function. I want you to take this literally: Negativity causes the stress hormone cortisol to go up. Positivity causes it to go down. Every thought and emotion you think and feel has a physical effect on your body. Just as negative emotions put you in a "fight" or "flight" mode, positive thinking allows you to rest, relax, and recover. While you are resting, your body is using that time to repair cells, detox, and regulate hormones. If you are constantly stressed, from thinking negatively about yourself or feeling unable to cope with life circumstances happening to you or around you, your body doesn't have the time to recover and you age faster because your cells aren't being repaired, you accumulate toxins, and your hormones continue being imbalanced. You feel like you're just trying to get through each day alive and you fall into a pattern of bad habits that keeps you in a vicious cycle of self-medicating through maybe smoking, drinking, or my personal past favorite, Ben and Jerry's (Peanut Butter Cup, if you're wondering). Like Jim Carey said in *Ace Ventura, Pet Detective*, "I have exorcised the demons!" Now it's your turn, too.

Practicing Self Love

I talk to women. Lots and lots of women. The older women I talk to at my clinic often lack confidence in themselves. They are self-conscious that they are "getting old" and they feel like their bodies are slowly falling apart as they reminisce of when they were more youthful. Ironically, the younger women I talk to at my clinic also lack confidence in themselves. They are self-conscious of tiny details that most people would never even notice. They see imperfections, thanks to our society's impossible standards of female beauty.

If you don't love yourself, and by that, I mean love the essential you in you —eventually you'll find that everything else will begin to lose its shimmer for you. Why? Because it is your spirit which looks out at the world and loves, feels, and embraces. If you cannot cherish yourself then you may lose the ability to show love for others as well. By loving yourself, I'm not talking so much about appearance-wise, but loving your heart, soul, drive, dreams, ambition, goodness and wisdom—all those inner qualities you now know are rare and beautiful. All it takes is motivation and a positive attitude to make big changes that will help you rescue your health and improve the body and mind.

Breaking bad habits is a monumental undertaking and an achievement to be mighty proud of, no matter how "small" these changes might seem. Choosing to eat a more nutrient-dense diet or give up a favorite food that's not-so-good for you will take giving up a creature comfort that is giving you something that you've been counting on to get you through hard days, hard times, or simply lift the mood. And to most women going through menopause, mood can make or break a whole day.

No matter what your body looks like now, you need to think about how you got there. Life is a war-zone. With stress from trying to balance career and family, going through pregnancy and childbirth, unfortunate events such as loss of a loved one, or dealing with other very difficult issues, we are only human and can only do so much and can only handle things the best we can. Stress can cause bad eating habits as a way of dealing with it, leading to weight gain. Remember that you have been through a lot, so thank yourself for pulling through. Thank your body for all it's been through and for carrying you through all this intact and for all the places its carried you that brought you joy, maybe children, love, life, loss, and for allowing you to enjoy so many days full of positivity, light, and laughter. These days are not over but are only stepping stones towards what is to come: A reinvention of yourself. A stronger, beautiful woman with the gift of acceptance and the ability to share her talents and wisdom with others. It's time to be the star others look up to.

There are many ways to try to feel more of a sense of love and acceptance toward growing older, even if that means a little extra padding, laugh lines, and graying hair. Life is short, ladies, and look how many years have gone by so quickly. You deserve to have a beautiful life and be happy while you're here. Let's make that happen *now*.

Great Ways to Love Yourself during Menopause (and Raise Your Happiness Quotient)

1. **Think about what you absolutely love about being an older (and much wiser) woman**

One of the best ways to enjoy gratitude for getting older is to really think hard about how much life improves as we age. We all idealize our teens and twenties, but were you nearly as happy with yourself then as you are now? About 99% of older women say they feel relieved they no longer worry about what everybody thinks about them.

Now, write down a bunch of things you love about being older on little strips of colored paper as you think of them. Put them folded or scrunched decoratively into a big, decorative jar or fishbowl. On bad days, when you are body or age-shaming yourself, reach in and pick out something that will help you keep your eyes on becoming a better future self instead of dwelling on the past.

Some things to be proud of as you get older may include:

- Knowing that if there's no beauty inside, it doesn't exist on the outside either. Being humble and grateful adds to a woman's beauty.
- Having wisdom. Older women's knowledge and experience means they make better decisions.
- Goodbye to drama. In your youth, you may have been drawn to the dramatic, but today, it's not worth your time. Your life is no longer a soap opera. You have peace.
- Not having to feel apologetic about spending less time doing things you don't want to. Your time is valuable and you aren't going to waste it on only making others happy and forgetting about yourself.
- Having the courage to stand up for yourself. With age comes a sense of fearlessness.
- You have more time to spend with loved ones. Mothers often lack time. Grandmothers make up for it. You can spend all the time and money you want spoiling your dog, too.
- Knowing who you are, not having to prove yourself.
- Having more stability, knowing where you are going in life.

In short, don't waste one more second of your beautiful life on self-doubt. You cannot just "wait around" for confidence and self-belief to happen. These feelings aren't handed to you. Like every valuable thing, they must be worked hard for.

2. Choose your Cheerleaders

Surround yourself with people who genuinely like you and cheer you on every day. The last thing you want around is a person who does not wish you well in life. You know this type. They're grouchy and eager to put the subject back on themselves. Even if you say one thing about yourself, and no matter what good things you do, they'll give you reasons why there's nothing so special about that or *anything you do.* Get away from these people as fast as you can—as if they have something contagious that makes you age 80 years overnight—because sister, THEY kind of do—it's a disease called narcissism (or heartlessness).

A circle of good female friends are heaven for the soul. If you have old friends who have known you since you were a girl, you're in luck. These kinds of friends may live far away and you may not see or talk to them for years but they'll still know you at your little girl soul-core, the thing in us that never changes and only grows more layers. One thing you can do to armor yourself against loneliness, worries about aging, or depression is to surround yourself with healthy female friendships. If you've been busy with career and/or family and have not been cultivating your friendship garden for some time, try getting involved in some crafts classes, quilting groups, painting classes, swimming classes, Yoga or Pilates classes, or a reading club. Often, there's other women there who'd love a new friend to talk with and to do things with— in fact, they might be there just to meet someone like you!

3. Don't neglect exercise

Exercise not only lifts mood and helps fight depression but forms of exercise such as strength training can also help you build more fat-burning muscle (in a feminine way), kick menopausal weight gain to the curb and lean your body out, which will make you feel like you want to go anywhere, even to the grocery store, to show it off. Middle-aged hottie in aisle seven! Check out that confident, sexy momma who knows what she wants! Through regular exercise, you will increase your willpower and dedication, and with all those happy brain chemicals being released every time you work out, you'll feel more positive, think more clearly, and realize that life is only just getting started.

4. Make sleep a major priority

There's no treatment, cream, or injection better than sleep for the skin, models will tell you. Getting high-quality sleep and lots of it helps to balance hormones, boosts mood by allowing ample time for neurotransmitter production and regulation (happy brain chemicals), and it also increases the amount of time we spend in slow wave sleep, a stage of sleep right after REM sleep when we burn fat, heal wounds, perform collagen synthesis, and all kinds of essentials for a menopausal woman's overall health and happiness quotient. We need as many slow wave sleep cycles we can get in order to experience the kind of cellular chemical reactions that result in better health and beautiful skin. In fact, we need four to five cycles of slow wave sleep a night. This can only be achieved by going to bed early and getting 7 to 9 (yes, *nine*) hours of sleep a night. Sleep deprivation results in a build-up of free radicals and superoxides in the brain, which means brain cells become damaged [18], hormones become imbalanced, your body becomes inflamed, your metabolism is affected, and you're more likely to gain weight [19].

5. Self-Pamper Your Way to Self-Love

Self-Pampering is a way to tell yourself you love yourself with actions, not words. It is also a great way to stay happy and healthy. For women going through menopause, it is highly essential to take time for yourself as your body is undergoing a lot of changes. Taking time out for you, no matter who needs what from you, is what it will take if you're struggling with menopause.

When menopause hits, many women are not used to giving themselves proper self-care but this is when it becomes essential. With the more severe symptoms like insomnia and depression, women just simply can't continue as they did. Something has got to give! At this stage, good self-care is non-negotiable.

Self-care is not selfish. We need to look after ourselves first and then, and only then, give to others. It is like when you are in an airplane during the safety demonstration and the flight attendant tells you to put on your own oxygen mask first and only then, can you help others with theirs. It is common sense [20].

Self-Pampering Idea #1. Make your home fit for a queen (that's you!)

While you're working hard on loving yourself and your body, why not take a year or so to make your home the one you always wanted, richly decorated with all your favorite pictures, colors, sights, and deliciously scented aromas you love wafting from diffusers and organic candles. Comfort comes from a clean, uncluttered home that reflects who you really are. You deserve a home that you want to kick back in, look around at your space and feel content and proud of.

Self-Pampering Idea #2. Get fridge fancy

Ever heard of the saying, "Whole Foods, whole paycheck?" Well, sometimes it's good to splurge. Clean out your fridge and pantry over the weekend and replace all the cheap, processed, unhealthy foods (pretty much anything that comes in a box or can) that are causing inflammation in your body and replace with fresh, organic, crisp vegetables and fruit, nuts and seeds, and high-quality cuts of meat and seafood. Make it look like a green goddess slid down from Heaven on a rainbow of fruits and vegetables, landing in your kitchen. Splurge on some pricier items that you would normally feel guilty about. Spend some time in the kitchen over the weekend preparing delicious dishes that nourish your mind, body and soul and enjoy the fanciest TV dinner ever while binge-watching chick flicks.

Self-Pampering Idea #3. Enjoy a digital detox

It's hard to imagine surviving an entire weekend without a phone or computer. But if you want to pamper yourself at home, especially after a busy week, the weekend is a perfect time for a digital detox. Excessive screen time can not only lead to headaches, eye strain, neck pain, and sleeping problems, but it can also make you feel stressed out. The average American spends more than half of their awake time staring at a screen. Turn off all the sounds on your gadgets, don't check your emails, stay off social media, and disconnect to reconnect with yourself. Everything can wait until Monday. Like, literally.

Did You Know?
Although studies are not fully convincing, there may also be some skin damage from the blue light emitted by phones and computer screens. Also think that if your computer screen is by a window, you are exposed to UVAs. It is well known that UVAs are damaging the skin. So, a break from your phone and computer is important!

Practicing Stress Reduction

Another form of self-love is putting yourself in a place where you feel like you have balance in everyday life. One problem I used to have is that I had a difficult time monitoring my stress level. I would never turn down an opportunity so my task list kept growing and it left me little to no time for myself. Eventually I found myself burnt out, depressed, and falling into bad diet habits which made me feel even worse. I couldn't concentrate, my memory was shot, my hormones were out of whack, and my kids thought I was turning into a MOMster. Stress got the best of me.

Stress is the body's reaction to harmful situations, whether they're real or perceived. Stress is also a state of mind. I know, you probably hate me for saying that but it's true. Stress starts in the brain. Whatever we sense from the environment (a dog barking, a car driving towards us, etc) gets sent to different parts of our brain. The amygdala, the emotional and impulsive part of our brain, decides whether or not we are being threatened and lets our body know how to respond quickly. Another part of our brain, the cerebral cortex, tries to rationalize whether or not we are in as great a danger as we think we are. Once the amygdala and cerebral cortex have made a decision together, they pass the message on to the hypothalamus, which then sends signals to two other structures: the pituitary gland, and the adrenal medulla. These short term responses are produced by The Fight or Flight Response via the sympathomedullary pathway (SAM). Long term stress is regulated by the hypothalamic pituitary-adrenal (HPA) system.

Cortisol can be bossy. It's a very powerful hormone in the body and if it gets out of control, it can throw other hormones off balance, too. Cortisol is produced by the adrenal glands. The adrenal glands also produce small amounts of estrogen, progesterone, and testosterone. They tend to pick up production more around the time of perimenopause and menopause, when the ovaries are slowing down. If chronic stress is a problem, the adrenal glands are too busy making more cortisol to deal with it, and less estrogen, progesterone, and testosterone are produced. That means perimenopause and menopause hits even harder.

Modern times make it hard to avoid stress, so we just have to deal with it by learning how to manage it.

Great Ways to Slow Down and Stress Less

1. Breath Focus

This is a simple yet powerful technique that you can do anywhere by taking long, slow deep breaths (also known as belly or abdominal breathing). As you breathe, focus on your breath and let all other sounds fade into the background. Gently redirect any thoughts or sensations to the simple exercise of breathing. Sometimes it helps to count each breath, up to ten and then start over again.

2. Balanced Exercise

Yes, exercise can be a real stress-reliever. However, this may sound counterintuitive, but too much exercise can actually make your stress level go up, not down. Excess exercise can cause your cortisol levels to rise, which makes it difficult to get a good night's sleep and makes you feel unrefreshed when you wake up in the morning. This is when most people reach for the coffee mug to start some spark but with all that caffeine, you end up feeling wired yet tired. So how do you find out what the best type and amount of exercise is best for you? By following these tips:

- My first tip is to pay attention to how you feel after you exercise. Do you feel peacefully tired but rejuvenated soon after? If so, repeat what you did the next time you work out or bump it up just a little. Or, if you feel worn out for several hours after exercise, it probably means that you should take it easier next time and hold off on increasing your activity.
- My second tip is to learn which types of exercise you enjoy doing. Exercise can truly be anything, whether it's walking, dancing, biking, or playing Frisbee. If you see exercise as a chore then you are not going to do it for very long and it could even stress you out thinking about having to do it.

3. Body Work

Getting a massage, acupuncture, acupressure, or simply stretching can provide you with some much needed time for yourself and help restore you both mentally and physically. Don't feel guilty about doing something special only for you. You have to take care of yourself before others because if you're worn out then you won't have the energy for anyone else.

4. Social Support

Talking to good friends is one of the best forms of stress reduction. It's like going to a counseling session without having to pay for one. Surround yourselves with friends who know you, who have the best intentions, and open yourself up to them by sharing not only all of the good things happening in your life but also your present worries. They'll feel good that you trust them enough to be vulnerable with them.

CHAPTER 5

CLEAN YOUR BODY: SYNTHETIC HORMONES AND POST-BIRTH CONTROL SYNDROME

"The 'science' behind hormone replacement therapy has put women on a medically engineered, press-fueled, big pharma funded roller coaster ride." — Willow Bay

The manufacturing of estrogen pills from the urine of pregnant horses sparked a huge revolution for women beginning in the 1940's. For many years, practitioners regularly prescribed this synthetic (man-made) hormone to women going through menopause. Women were told that the treatment, called hormone replacement therapy (HRT) would help not only with bothersome hot flashes, night sweats and vaginal dryness, but would also protect them from a multitude of health problems, including heart disease. However, in 2002, a national study called the Women's Health Initiative, asserted that the specific regimen of synthetic estrogen and progestin (a synthetic form of progesterone) being used by millions of women did not protect against heart disease and stroke and actually did more harm than good. In fact, the results showed that women taking the hormones had an increased risk for breast cancer, stroke, heart attack, and blood clots.

- Premarin: estrogen made from pregnant horse urine. It is a natural estrogen but does not have the molecular structure of human estrogen and therefore can have different effects on the body.
- Provera, Aygestin, and Megace. Synthetic forms of progesterone (progestins).
- PremPro: combination of Premarin and Provera. It is the most commonly used form of conventional HRT.

An important limitation of the Women's Health Initiative was that it only tested synthetic hormones. This means that the molecular structure of these synthetic hormones does not match our own, so our body may react to them and relieve symptoms but may also suffer from negative side effects as well. Because of the limitation in the study, we didn't learn about the safety and effectiveness of other hormone formulations such as bio-identical progesterone and estrogen, which do match the molecular structure of our own hormones, different delivery methods such as medication taken by mouth or applied to the skin, or the combination of hormones with natural supplements such as diindolylmethane (DIM). The end of the study left a lot of unanswered questions.

Note: I offer hormone replacement therapy in my clinic. The decision to start someone on it is on a case-by-case basis with a well-researched assessment of potential harms and benefits. I do not prescribe synthetic hormones. I only prescribe bio-identical hormones.

Why can synthetic hormones cause problems?

Your ovarian hormones are estradiol, progesterone, and testosterone. They have many benefits, not only for reproduction, but also for metabolism, bone and muscle health, and mood. Your body recognizes them and accepts them as part of yourself. In contrast, the molecular structures in synthetic hormone medications to treat menopause and other conditions, including the birth control pill, are not recognized in the same way and because of this, they can make you feel crummy and negatively impact your health. These "fake" hormones such as levonorgestrel and ethinylestradiol, have different effects in the body. Levonorgestrel, a synthetic form of progesterone, has been linked with depression and anxiety [21], hair loss, weight gain, bloating, and even symptoms of blood sugar problems. Ethinylestradiol, the synthetic form of estrogen, has been linked with blood clots, liver damage, and cancer of the uterus [22].

The Birth Control Pill: Friend and Foe

Far back in history, the women's main job was to produce offspring. The men went out hunting, gathering food for the family, and protecting them from danger. The woman cared for the young, often multiple, while continuing to breastfeed even though the child was old enough to run off to pick their own berries, or when they became pregnant again and their milk production dwindled down. But now we live in modern times. Most women wait until their thirties to become pregnant, focus on their careers, hope to have one boy and one girl, and decide to stop breastfeeding their baby at age one because that's what they were told to do in their parenting manuals.

Currently, the average desired family size in the U.S. is two children and the average attained family size is two-and-a-half. To achieve this family size, a woman must use contraceptives for roughly three decades [23], most commonly through hormonal methods. That means for around thirty years, a woman is put into a chemically-induced menopausal state, preventing her ovaries from releasing eggs, preventing her body to prepare for a fertilized egg, and changing her cervical mucous to make it difficult for sperm to pass through the cervix and find an egg. These hormones in her birth control pills are made in a laboratory, often from the urine of pregnant horses.

In the United States, there are currently 61 million women in their childbearing years (age 15-44) and about sixty-seven percent primarily use hormonal methods of birth control [23]. The pill has been the most common method of birth control and has been since 1965, five years after it gained FDA approval and fell into the hands of the general public. Before then, people relied on condoms, spermicide, the "pull-out method," abstinence, and listen to this...Ancient Egyptian women used vaginal suppositories made from cotton, dates, honey, and fermented acacia.

Thoughts of birth control enter our minds at a young age. Sex education is taught in middle school and the children are taught about various forms of contraception. There are plenty of hormonal birth control options out there. Don't want to have to take a pill every day? Get a shot every three months instead. Is a period going to ruin that beautiful beach getaway you've been planning? Take a pill that only gives you a period every three months. Do you just hate having a period altogether? Take a pill 365 days a year and never experience those annoying periods again. Does your partner blame arguments on your PMS? There's a pill for that, too. No more PMS. Take some fake hormones and you'll have a happy husband and harmonious household.

These conveniences, however, come with a price. IUDs may cause pelvic inflammatory disease and ovarian cysts. Depo-Provera shots may induce osteoporosis. Birth control pills may cause hormonal turmoil, accelerated aging, increased risk of heart disease and cancer, and also contribute to weight gain, blood clots especially in smokers, decreased bone density, impaired sex drive, gallbladder disease, and depression. These are things that were not talked about in middle school sex ed. Most women don't find out about them until years after they stopped using the pill or other methods of contraception. Or, at least they didn't think it would happen to them. More and more women are faced with hormonal problems that weren't even related to their sex hormones. They frequently encounter thyroid problems, especially hypothyroidism (low thyroid). Birth control pills deplete selenium, zinc and the amino acid tyrosine from our bodies. These are all vitamins and minerals that are necessary for proper thyroid function! Excess hormones from birth control can stress the liver since it must work harder to break them down for elimination. This can lead to inflammation and poor immune function, triggering autoimmune disorders, which means the body is basically attacking itself.

Breaking Up with Hormonal Birth Control

Your doctor may have told you that birth control pills can delay menopause. However, that is not true and if anything, they can contribute to early menopause [24]. Many women are also put on the pill to treat symptoms of menopause. As you read earlier, synthetic hormones come with a lot of risks. Stopping the pill is your decision to make. If you do take that leap, you may want to consult with your medical provider first.

Post-Birth Control Syndrome

Something more and more women are going to start hearing about is Post-Birth Control Syndrome. If you have never heard of it and have taken birth control pills, I strongly recommend you read Dr. Jolene Brighten's book, "Beyond the Pill." Birth control pills can prevent unwanted pregnancies, but make no mistake, they do so by flooding your body with chemicals that change the way your brain communicates with your ovaries and reproductive system in order to either stop ovulation (progestin-estrogen pills) or thicken cervical mucus so much as to make it difficult for sperm to enter (progestin only), where they could fertilize an egg and make you pregnant.

Some women feel okay while on birth control pills. Personally, they made me sick to my stomach, depressed, and I also weighed the most I ever had. That doesn't happen with everyone and a few women just glide right through without any side effects. However, one serious but not widely known side effect that doesn't occur until later is Post-Birth Control Syndrome, which typically happens within 4 to 6 months of stopping the pill.

Symptoms of Post-Birth Control Syndrome

- **Amenorrhea:** complete loss of periods or just mild spotting instead of a full period. In fact, for some 3 to 6% of women, their period *never returns.*
- **Irregular/Unpredictable periods:** heavy bleeding, short cycles, or very painful periods with severe cramping.
- **Hormone disorders:** thyroid disorders such as hypothyroidism, infertility, and breast tenderness.

- **Hair loss:** birth control pills cause the hair to move out of the growing phase and into the resting phase too quickly, which is called telogen effluvium.
- **Acne:** many women go on the pill to heal acne, only to find going off the pill causes worse symptoms than before.
- **Mood swings and disorders:** Anxiety, increased episodes of crying, and depression are just a few side effects of hormonal changes caused by going off hormonal birth control.
- **Hormonal changes.** These can include infertility, hypothyroidism, HPA-axis dysfunction, and other changes you may not have experienced while on the pill.
- **Weight gain/difficulty losing weight.** Weight gain is common with the pill/hormonal birth control and can make losing weight quite difficult even once one goes off the pill (until you fully detoxify the body).
- **Digestive issues** such as bloating, gas, or diarrhea.

Post-Birth Control Syndrome Detox

Your liver is your main detox organ. That means it is responsible for moving synthetic hormones out of the body, especially when levels are too high. To help your liver to do this difficult task, it needs to be supported. Also, your intestinal tract needs to be functioning well so that hormones can be eliminated (no poop, no pass). Eating healthy, making sure you are having regular bowel movements, and supporting your liver are 3 major components of detoxing from synthetic hormones. I highly recommend you check out my program, "The 5-Day Detox", available at DoctorCarissa.com. This is a quick and easy-to-follow diet that will provide you with the right amount of anti-inflammatory foods, fiber and liver-supporting nutrients to help clean you out and help you get your hormones back into balance.

Non-Hormonal Birth Control Alternatives

I am not saying that women should never take hormonal birth control. There may be circumstances where the risk outweighs the benefit. One of the most concerning to women getting off the pill is obviously the risk of becoming pregnant. My mom's best friend stopped taking the pill because she thought she was in menopause and low and behold, nine months later a baby was born, 20 years after her last child.

My great-grandmother had 15 children, bless her. For me, three was plenty. For some, none is plenty. I have plenty of friends who are 100% content with being dog moms. Luckily, I know of some alternatives to birth control pills that I will share with you, in case you don't trust your ovaries right now.

Fertility Awareness Method

Men are fertile every single day. Women aren't. In fact, there are only six days that a woman is fertile during her monthly cycle. If you can avoid these days, you very likely won't get pregnant, unless there's some sort of immaculate conception happening. The Fertility Awareness Method, which means abstaining from sex or using a barrier method such as a condom during your fertile days, can be as effective as taking hormonal birth control when used perfectly. Of course, we aren't all perfect, so the typical failure rate using Fertility Awareness Method ranges from 2-23% [25].

Pros: It does not mess up your hormones, put toxic chemicals into your body, or cause unpleasant side effects or negatively impact your health.

Cons: You have to track your ovulation and abstain from sex or use a barrier method on your fertile days. It does not protect against sexually transmitted diseases unless you use a barrier method. It has a high rate of failure.

Barrier Methods

Male condoms, female condoms, diaphragms, sponges, and cervical caps all prevent sperm from entering your uterus. These are sometimes used with spermicide.

Pros: Barrier methods (without spermicide) do not mess up your hormones, put toxic chemicals into your body, do not require a prescription, and are widely available. Condoms protect against sexually transmitted diseases.

Cons: Barrier methods may make sex less pleasurable, can be distracting during sex, and come with a higher failure rate (male condom 18%, female condom 28%, diaphragm without spermicide 12%, cervical cap without spermicide 8%) than some other methods [25]. Some products may cause skin irritation.

Copper Intrauterine Device (IUD)

The copper IUD has been around for a long time and is a small device made of copper and plastic that is inserted through a woman's cervix and into her uterus to prevent pregnancy by impairing sperm motility and changing the uterine lining so that a fertilized egg cannot implant and develop.

Pros: Set it and forget it. Once the IUD is inserted into place, you don't have to think about it for 10 years or more. It is highly effective with a failure rate of only 0.6% [25]. It won't mess up your hormones either.

Cons: It can be unpleasant during insertion, can cause heavy periods, and there's a small risk of the IUD coming out. It may increase the risk of infection or copper toxicity.

Withdrawal or Pull-Out Method

The oldest method of birth control, the withdrawal or pull-out method is exactly as it sounds: your partner pulls out his penis and ejaculates outside of your vagina.

> **Pros**: You don't need to do anything except hope your partner pulls out on time.

> **Cons**: The typical failure rate is pretty high at 28% [25] and you can't have sex multiple times because sperm remains in your partner's penis after the first ejaculation and can end up in your vagina.

Deciding on Hormone Replacement Therapy

Perimenopause and menopause are not disease states, however, plenty of women don't feel healthy during this time and it's important to have options. Any type of medication, whether hormones or drugs such as antidepressants, blood pressure and cholesterol medications, may result in unanticipated adverse effects, so every woman's decision to use them needs to be a personal, well-researched assessment of their potential risks and benefits.

The most natural and safest approach to treating symptoms of menopause is the right combination of diet and exercise. That's why you're reading this book, right? Many women have been able to relieve their symptoms of menopause and lose the extra weight it brings by using my protocol. If that's not enough to help you feel better, that's when it's time to consider adding hormone replacement therapy.

CHAPTER 6
CLEAN YOUR HOME: REDUCING TOXINS IN YOUR ENVIRONMENT

"We stopped cleaning our houses with lemon water and vinegar like our mothers did, and we clean with chemicals. We're breathing chemicals, and then everyone wonders why cancer is the biggest killer." — Suzanne Somers

As women, we are constantly bombarded by toxic chemicals in our environment and the food we eat. From the moment we shower, brush our teeth, and apply lotions and makeup, to the time we commute from work back home during 5 o'clock traffic, we are exposed to a conveyer line of chemicals. Our home is meant to be a clean space but it is one of the most toxic environments we spend our time in. Keeping our homes looking neat and tidy often means making them "dirtier." Sure, if we wipe our countertops with cleaning spray, they may look clean but what you don't see is a film of chemicals left behind, which end up on our skin and in our food. And that fresh smell we all love? It is none other than chemical fumes clouding our lungs and being sent straight to our brains. My cleaning lady came to me one day with concerns about acne. She said since she started her cleaning business, her skin broke out in pimples and her periods became very heavy, sometimes coming twice in one month. It only made sense. She was being exposed to toxic cleaning products all day, every day, which were interfering with her hormones. I told her that she should charge a little more and offer an organic cleaning service, that it would be good for both her and her customers.

Exposure to toxic chemicals is the real deal. I once heard a radio ad for a weight loss program that promised the use of no medications, no counting calories, and you could apparently lose up to 30 pounds in 30 days (which, by the way, I don't actually recommend to anyone unless you are highly supervised by a medical provider). I wanted to know how their weight loss program worked. So, I contacted my friend, Virginia, who had been a patient of theirs, and she shared the diet plan that they gave her with me. Part of their plan was to throw out all shampoo, conditioner, lotion, and pretty much every other products the skin comes in contact with and replace them with products from a provided list. Through my research, I discovered that this entire weight loss program was based on one confining principle: Toxic chemicals are metabolism blockers and if you avoid them, your hormones will become better balanced which will fix your metabolism and you'll lose weight.

Pollution, chemicals in our food, chemicals in our cosmetics, even hidden toxins such as candles burning in your home (the majority of candles contain Paraffin, a sludge waste product from the petroleum industry that releases carcinogenic chemicals when burned).... These toxic chemicals we are exposed to are called "endocrine disruptors" because they interfere with our endocrine system, which is the collection of glands that produce hormones. Endocrine disruptors work by blocking the synthesis, transport, binding action, or metabolism of natural blood-borne hormones. They trick our bodies into thinking they are hormones, preventing the healthier effects of our true hormones. They can convince our bodies that there is too much of a hormone, leading to symptoms of having too much of that hormone even when it may actually be lacking.

Estrogen Disruptors. Also known as "xenoestrogens", estrogen disruptors are chemicals that temporarily or permanently alter the feedback loops in the brain, pituitary, thyroid, and ovaries by mimicking the effects of estrogen and triggering their specific receptors. They may also bind to hormone receptors and block the action of natural hormones. Being exposed to xenoestrogens may lead to estrogen dominance, which may not only make women feel terrible (breast tenderness, bloating, anxiety, etc) but is also associated with an increased risk of breast cancer, ovarian cysts, uterine fibroids, infertility and miscarriages.

Androgen Disruptors. These are endocrine disrupting chemicals that raise testosterone (an androgen hormone) in women but lower it in men. Women with PCOS have been found to have higher levels of bisphenol A (BPA) in their bodies. Boys exposed to (yes, even from that seemingly innocent swimming pool in the backyard) have been found to have lower levels of testosterone.

Common Sources of Endocrine Disruptors:

- Plastics
- Food: Meats containing hormones and any food with pesticide residue
- Cosmetics and toiletries
- Cleaning products
- Nail polish and nail polish remover
- Water (chlorine and chlorine byproducts)
- Birth control pills
- Perfumes and fragrances
- Automobile exhaust
- Cigarette smoke

There is no safe level of exposure to endocrine disruptors because they can be stored in our bodies, coined by the term "bioaccumulation." Bioaccumulation is the gradual buildup of chemicals and it happens when your body absorbs chemicals faster than it can eliminate them.
Poor liver function and sleep quality can affect the way we eliminate endocrine disruptors from our bodies. The liver is our main detoxifying organ, which means that a malfunctioning liver means less detoxing and a buildup up of toxins.

It's Time for Chores

Put on your cute little apron, lady, because it's time to do a little cleaning. Now that you get the idea of toxic chemicals that affect your hormone health and the unknown safety of GMOs, let's get dirty. We are going to clean up the three most toxic rooms in your house: Kitchen, bathroom, and laundry room. Grab a large, heavy-duty garbage bag and go from room to room in your home and stuff every product we're going to discuss, every product that contains the chemicals we're about to talk about, into the bag. Use gloves. Better yet, tongs. If that's too big a step, at least get rid of anything that's marked "Danger" or "Poison" on the label. Please. And while you're at it, make a list of what needs to be replaced. Then, take a deep breath and say good-bye once and for all to your old life. Say hello to your happy little hormones and a better you.

Note: If the idea of tossing everything is too overwhelming, or cost is prohibitive, set a goal of replacing one item per week or month until you have replaced everything.

Kitchen Clean Up

Your kitchen is supposed to be one of the cleanest areas of your home. After all, this is where you prepare food, right? The problem is, most people don't realize that there are far more dangers being exposed to toxic chemicals than there are getting food poisoning. A friend of mine was shocked when she came to my house and saw that my newly renovated kitchen was comprised of wooden countertops. "But the bacteria!" she exclaimed. Well guess what?.. Our family has been living with wooden countertops for five years and not one of us (family of seven) has suffered from food poisoning because of it, and might I add, we don't use commercial antibacterial sprays. Why don't we use them? Because they aren't good for humans and they aren't much better than a bottle of ordinary white vinegar. I'll show you the proof shortly.

Cookware

Avoid all kinds of toxic cookware. The most toxic, by far, is non-stick cookware. Close runners up are aluminum cookware or those speckled baking dishes. The more toxic your body is overall, the less chance you have of eliminating specific toxins from the body, like excess estrogen. Safe cookware equals stainless steel, cast iron, glass, ceramic, or copper only.

Food Prep and Storage

Plastic. If plastic is bad for the environment, it only makes sense that it's also bad to store our food in it, right? The problem with plastic is that it contains harmful chemicals that may seep into our food, especially when heated, and can affect our hormones (remember that the next time you leave a plastic water bottle in a hot car). Two major chemicals to watch out for are phthalates (used to soften plastics) and bisphenol A (BPA), which is used to make very hard, shatterproof plastic (it usually has #7 on the bottom) and is also found in the lining of canned foods and beverages. Although numerous studies have found BPA to cause reproductive harm and cancer, it is still legal in most of the United States (but banned in some other countries). Just because a plastic food container is phthalate and BPA-free doesn't mean it's entirely safe. Of the 80,000 chemicals produced and used in the U.S. today, the Environmental Protection Agency has required testing on only 200, leaving a lot of uncertainty over their safety and long-term effects.

Aluminum is one of the most abundant metals on Earth and is naturally found in small amounts in water and food. However, cooking with it at high temperatures (like when you bake a potato) or with acidic foods (like tomatoes), can cause high amounts of aluminum to pass into your food. Some research has suggested that excessive consumption of aluminum from it leaching into food has extreme health risk effects [26]. Although some studies have found it to be safe, I recommend avoiding it to be on the safe side.

Styrofoam. You would be doing the environment and your health a favor by reducing use of Styrofoam containers. Unfortunately, some recyclers won't take foam containers because they're so light and the profit in recycling is calculated by weight. That means Styrofoam containers blow away and often end up in the ocean. In addition to harming marine life, Environmental Protection Agency and International Agency for Research on Cancer state that styrene possibly causes cancer. Some research suggests that styrene can leach out of foam food containers and cups when food or drinks are hot. Think about that the next time you order take-out for dinner.

You can recognize styrene foam by looking for the number 6 inside the recycling symbol.

Silicone rubber does not react with food or beverages, or produce any hazardous fumes and appears to be safe. So far, no safety problems have been reported but personally I avoid silicone altogether because I don't think enough research has been done on it since it's a newer product. Maybe stick to silicone kitchen tools, such as spatulas, and avoid bakeware if you're concerned. And if you buy silicone products, make sure you get good quality ones that don't contain any filler, which may contain toxic chemicals. You can test it by pinching and twisting a flat surface to see if white shows through – if so, filler has been used.

Now that you know which materials are safe or possibly unsafe, I recommend you throw out these items:

- Plastic wrap
- Aluminum foil
- Plastic food storage bags
- Plastic food containers
- Plastic cups and water bottles
- Styrofoam cups
- Plastic baby bottles

And replace with these items:

- Reusable glass water bottles
- Reusable stainless steel bottles
- Glass food storage containers
- Glass Mason jars
- Lead-free ceramic food storage containers
- Glass baby bottles

Dishwasher Detergent

Dishwasher detergent can contain bleach, artificial fragrance, dyes, and a whole host of chemicals that are known to cause adverse health effects including respiratory issues, hormone imbalances, and even cancer.

Non-Toxic Dishwasher Detergents:

- Seventh Generation dishwasher detergent packs. I find they work just as well and are not too expensive.
- My #2 pick: Honest Company auto dishwasher detergent gel, free & clear

Hand Soap

Many hand soaps on store shelves are antibacterial. There are several problems with this. First, antibacterial hand soaps are no more effective than regular soap and water for killing disease-causing germs, according to the Centers for Disease Control. Second, antibacterial hand soaps are more expensive than regular hand soaps. Third, antibacterial hand soaps kill the healthy bacteria on your hands, which can make antibiotics less effective in the fight against new strains of bacteria, called superbugs.

Hand soap can contain toxic chemicals that may interfere with hormones, whether it is antibacterial or not. Even hand soaps labelled as "natural" commonly contain toxic ingredients because there are no federal regulations stipulating criteria for personal care products labeled as "natural."

Non-Toxic Hand Soaps:

- Dr. Bronner's Pure-Castile Hand Soap
- Seventh Generation Hand Wash

Furniture Cleaner

Dust... It's everywhere and it's not going away. Dust contains mostly shed human skin, animal hair if you have pets, decomposing insects, plant pollen, and even lead and arsenic. Considering it's not only gross and chronic exposure may lead to allergies, it's no wonder we want our home to pass the white glove test at all times.

Personally, I prefer not to use furniture cleaner at all. A microfiber cloth is the greenest possible way that you can dust your home, but sometimes you need something more. Most furniture cleaners contain toxic chemicals that you breathe in, which are "no bueno". According to the Environmental Working Group's Guide to Healthy Cleaning, some of the most hazardous ingredients in furniture cleaners include:

- C10-12 Alkane/Cycloalkane
- C12-20 Isoparaffin
- Cyclotetrasiloxane
- Petroleum Distillates
- Petroleum Gases
- Pthalates
- Sodium salts such as sodium borate

Non-Toxic Furniture Cleaner:

DIY Furniture Cleaner Recipe

1 cup water
½ cup vinegar
2 TBSP oil (coconut or olive are my top choices)
10 drops lemon essential oil (optional)
5 drops cedarwood essential oil (optional)

1. Pour water and vinegar into spray bottle.
2. Add oil and essential oils.
3. Cover bottle and shake well.

Antibacterial Cleaners

Antibacterial cleaners classified by law as pesticides and their germ--killing claims are specific and limited. In fact, some don't even claim to kill E. coli, one of the most commonly feared food-borne bacteria.

Their germ-killing ingredients aren't so good for humans or the kitchen, either: Labels include warnings about fumes and contact with skin or eyes, the importance of rinsing food-contact surfaces after use, and potential damage to common materials. Considering white distilled vinegar reduces bacteria by 99.9%, without carrying dangerous warning labels, it makes sense to skip modern antibacterial cleaners and revert back to grandma's tried and true cleaning solution: vinegar solution. You can use it to clean food surfaces (hey, it is vinegar after all), the inside of your fridge, and the windows.

Non-Toxic Antibacterial Spray:

Vinegar Solution (one-part white vinegar with one-part water)

Glass Cleaner

Most glass cleaners contain one or more of these harmful ingredients:

- Ammonia
- Butyl cellosolve, a glycol ether (also known as 2-butoxyethanol, 2-butoxyethanol acetate or Ethylene glycol monobutyl ether)
- Phthalates

Non-Toxic Glass Cleaner:

Vinegar Solution (one-part white vinegar with one-part water)

Tip: Annoyed by streaks on glass? Streaks that remain after cleaning glass with vinegar may be due to a waxy residue from previous glass cleaning products. Mix one-part rubbing alcohol with 20-parts water and remove any buildup before cleaning standard glass with vinegar.

Toilet Cleaner

You would think that because it goes into the toilet, you won't come into contact with it. However, even just breathing the fumes when pouring it into the bowl may be harmful.

Non-Toxic Toilet Cleaners:

- Seventh Generation Toilet Bowl Natural Cleaner
- Earth Friendly Products ECOS Toilet Cleaner

Bathroom Clean Up

The bathroom is a dirty place but right now I want you to forget about cleaning the toilet or bathtub. Instead, let's focus on the heap of cosmetics and toiletries you are probably hoarding. I'm sure you've been meaning to throw out all those half-used bottles of facial creams that didn't work, the tiny hotel shampoo and conditioners you didn't want to leave behind, or the clumpy nail polish from the 1990's you thought you would use again one day. Let's clear the clutter and start fresh, shall we? While we are at it, we are going to not only clear your mind of the clutter, but we are also going to help clear your body from the toxic wasteland residing in your bathroom cabinets.

The "Dirty Dozen" 12 Toxic Ingredients in Hair, Skin, and Nail Products

- **Parabens.** Parabens are a whole family of chemicals (methylparabens, propylparabens, butylparabens, and ethylparabens) that help preserve shelf-life of products. They are endocrine disruptors that can mimic estrogen, throwing off our delicate hormonal balance. They've been linked to breast cancer, and since they act as a hormone disruptor they can lead to reproductive and fertility issues.

- **Phthalates.** Phthalates are a group of chemicals used to make plastics softer and more flexible. They are used in skincare products to help the ingredients stick to our skin. Phthalates can be extremely dangerous to children and several types have already been banned from children's products. They can be serious endocrine disruptors and even cause birth defects.

- **Sodium lauryl sulfate (SES) and sodium laureth sulfate (SLES).** These are used to create that luxurious lather effect that we all love. SLS and SLES are known to cause skin irritation and trigger different allergies, as well as weakening hair and causing hair loss. In similar news, if you suffer from whiteheads and blackheads, it could be as a result of using face and body care products that contain SLS.

- **PEG compounds like propylene glycol.** These are petroleum-based ingredients that are used as thickeners, solvents, softeners, and moisture-carriers. That's why they are commonly used in cosmetic cream bases. Some PEGs have been found to be generally safe for adults but not enough research has been done on children. I think it's best to just avoid them if you have kids around.

- **DEA/TEA/MEA:** Suspected carcinogens used as emulsifiers and foaming agents for shampoos, body washes, soaps. They may also disrupt your hormone balance.

- **Formaldehyde.** Formaldehyde and formaldehyde-releasing preservatives (FRP's) are used in many cosmetic products to help prevent bacteria growth. It is a known cancer-causing chemical and can also cause allergic skin reactions and harm the immune system. It is banned in some countries.

- **Triclosan.** This is an antibacterial chemical that has been banned since 2016 but check if it's still lingering in your cabinets. It disrupts hormones, weakens the immune system, has been associated with cancer, and can cause developmental problems in children.

- **Butylated hydroxytoluene (BHT).** This is a preservative used to extend shelf life and may be an endocrine disruptor. Some research has found it causes liver, kidney, and lung damage.

- **Silicone-derived emollients (such as dimethicone):** Used to make your hair and skin feel smooth, soft, and create a water barrier to trap in moisture. These don't biodegrade, which means they are bad for the environment. Questions remain about chronic toxicity or the consequences of bioaccumulation since they can be long-lived.

- **Coal Tar:** A known carcinogen banned in some countries, it is still used in the United States for dry skin, lice and dandruff shampoos.

- **Petrolatum (Petroleum, petroleum jelly, mineral oil).** Petrolatum may mimic estrogen in the body. In addition, petrolatum is often not fully refined in the US, which means it can be contaminated with toxic chemicals called polycyclic aromatic hydrocarbons (PAHs), which have been linked to cancer.

- **Fragrance.** Doesn't sound scary, right? But "fragrance" is considered a trade secret which means that companies don't have disclose what ingredients are inside. Often, the ingredients include tons of chemicals that can trigger allergies, disrupt hormones and cause reproductive and fertility issues.

More toxic ingredients to look out for:

- **Synthetic colors.** If you take a look at your product label and notice FD&C or D&C, they represent artificial colors. "F" represents food and "D&C" represents drug and cosmetics. These letters precede a color and number (e.g., D&C Red 27 or FD&C blue 1). These synthetic colors are derived from petroleum or coal tar sources. Synthetic colors possibly cause cancer and have been banned in some countries.

- **Toluene.** Derived from petroleum or coal tar sources, you may see benzene, toluol, phenylmethane, or methylbenzene on labels. Toluene is a paint thinner so you may see it in nail polish. Pregnant women should avoid it as it may cause developmental damage to her baby. It has also been linked to immune system toxicity.

- **Paraphenylenediamine (PPD).** This is the most common and most well-known component of hair dyes and has been associated with cancer and is a skin, eye, and lung irritant and allergen.

A note on lavender and tea tree oil: These have been found to have estrogen-like effects in the body. Yep, two of the most popular essential oils are also endocrine disruptors. If you're sad, you're not the only one. It's not easy being married to someone from the South of France and knowing all that lavender isn't good for my hormones.

Shampoo and Conditioner

Hair care products like shampoo and conditioner are highly engineered. They've been designed to lather up and leave your hair "squeaky clean," but that's not even that good for you! The chemicals in shampoo strip your hair of natural oils that are meant to be there to protect. That's why we have to condition our hair after we shampoo – to re-moisturize it without leaving it oily. Achieving the desired effect without using any harmful ingredients is nearly impossible and that's why many organic shampoos are not 100% pure. Now I am not going to tell you to withhold from washing your hair for one year like my husband did while backpacking in South America when he was in his 20's (although he said his curls looked shiny and amazing). But I do recommend checking your shampoo and conditioner bottles for the toxic ingredients and replacing them with some that don't.

Non-Toxic Shampoo and Conditioners:

- Avalon Organics Shampoo and Conditioner
- BeautyCounter Shampoo and Conditioner

Soap and Body Wash

Wash on, wash off? Showering is part of your everyday routine to keep your body clean, fresh, and smelling good. What if this simple habit was exposing you to harsh and potentially dangerous ingredients or chemicals? Your skin is the largest organ of your body and absorbs anything that you put onto it, including toxic chemicals that can harm you.

Non-Toxic Soap and Body Wash:

- Dr. Bronner's Pure Castile Soap
- Seven Minerals Pure Castile Soap

Lotions and Creams

One of the main ways your body acquires nutrients, other than eating, is through the skin. Your skin is your largest organ, 22 square feet on average, and 60% of the substances you put on it are eventually absorbed into the bloodstream. This semipermeable membrane allows us to absorb vitamins and minerals, but, unfortunately, it also absorbs harmful chemicals we put on it. Body washes can contain toxic chemicals that your skin is briefly exposed to. Just imagine how much more toxic chemicals your body absorbs when they are left on your skin for even longer periods of time, such as in the case of lotions and creams?

Non-toxic lotions and creams:

- Shea Moisture Lotion, Raw Shea Butter
- NOW Solutions Cocoa Butter Lotion

Makeup

Because needs can vary greatly when it comes to skin color, skin type, and skin concerns, I'll leave out my recommendations. I do suggest that you visit the Environmental Working Group's Skin Deep Guide (ewg.org/skindeep) to find out how safe your makeup products actually are.

Nail Polish and Removers

Take a whiff and you already know that nail polish and remover are packed with harmful chemicals.
Non-toxic nail polishes:

- Zoya Professional Lacquer
- Piggy Paint Nail Polish

Non-Toxic Nail Polish Removers:

- Mineral Fusion Nail Polish Remover
- Karma Organic Beauty Natural Soybean Nail Polish Remover

Deodorant

Walk into any organic market store and you'll find shelves stocked with "natural" deodorants, with labels boldly advertising that they're aluminum-free. This raises an important question: Does aluminum in deodorants cause breast cancer? The answer is no. There is no scientific evidence to support this idea. It's a myth and it has been debunked for quite some time. However, aluminum salts can be irritating to the skin, and there may be other ingredients in the deodorant that could cause harm.

Non-Toxic Deodorants:

- Thinksport Natural Deodorant
- Tom's of Maine Natural Deodorant

Toothpaste

The problem with toothpaste is that it contains fluoride, which is a controversial ingredient that in small amounts is beneficial for your teeth but in higher amounts causes toxicity. Just like with using aluminum cookware, your body can absorb some aluminum and store it, so there is a concern that little by little, the fluoride in our drinking water, toothpaste, and other sources build up and cause problems. My take on it is that you should either avoid it or make sure you rinse your mouth with water after you brush to avoid swallowing any.

Non-Toxic Toothpastes:

- Dr. Brite Mint Activated Charcoal Whitening Mineral Toothpaste
- Tom's of Maine Antiplaque & Whitening Toothpaste

Mouthwash

Do you remember those commercials that told you to suffer through your mouthwash routine? Well, a lot of us still suffer a daily morning war between burning swishes of mouthwash versus bad-breath-causing bacteria. While mouthwash *does* kill bacteria, it doesn't distinguish between harmful bacteria and the healthy bacteria that live in your mouth. Since antibacterial mouthwashes can wipe out every little organism living in your mouth and dry it out, your bad breath can get worse. In addition, mouthwashes sometimes contain chemicals that interfere with our hormone balance. The best way to keep your mouth smelling fresh is to brush, floss, and scrape your tongue at least twice a day – no mouthwash needed.
But if you're adamant about your morning gargle, there are some safe options.

Non-Toxic Mouthwashes:

- Dr. Brite Mouth Rinse
- DIY Mouthwash Recipe

1. 1 cup distilled water
2. 1 teaspoon baking soda
3. 1 teaspoon salt
4. 5 drops essential oil (peppermint or lemon are my faves)
5. Mix ingredients in a glass container and shake well. You'll have to shake with each use.

The Secret of Unsafe Sunscreen

I still remember the painful nights I endured during summers in Florida when I was a teenager. The consequences of slathering baby oil all over my skin were brutal. My hair was desiccated from Sun-In and lemon juice, hoping to achieve summer highlights that I couldn't have gotten otherwise because I wasn't allowed to bleach my hair. I was a sun worshipper. Years later, I found myself spraying SPF 70 on my kids while they occasionally gagged on the fumes. I thought I was doing the right thing applying sunscreen, until several more years later. I found out that sunscreen sprays may be unsafe and high SPF sunscreens may actually raise the risk of cancer.

The problem with sunscreen sprays is that they contain chemicals that can be harmful, especially towards hormones. Even the Food and Drug Administration (FDA) proposes that there are only two chemicals that we have enough safety information about to determine they are safe and effective and those are zinc oxide and titanium dioxide. So go into your bathroom and throw out sunscreen products that contain any of these 5 chemicals that carry the highest risk of toxicity (tip: avoid all the "O's" in sunscreen):

- Oxybenzone
- Octinoxate
- Homosalate
- Octisalate
- Octocrylene

The problem with high-SPF sunscreens (SPF over 50) according to the FDA is that they not only overpromise protection, they may also overexpose people to UVA rays and raise their risk of cancer (sunscreen only blocks UVB rays, fyi). Since high-SPF sunscreens contain higher concentrations of chemicals, they may have a greater effect on your hormones. So go into your bathroom and throw out sunscreen products with an SPF of 50 or higher.

Using a sunscreen should be a last resort. Wearing shorts, pants, and hats that shield your skin from the sun's UV rays can reduce your risk of burn by 27%. Planning your day around the sun, such as going outdoors in the early morning or late afternoon when the sun is lower in the sky can also help reduce sunburns.

Non-Toxic Sunscreens:

- Badger Active Natural Mineral Sunscreen Cream, Unscented, SPF 30
- Blue Lizard Australian Sunscreen, SPF 30

Laundry Room Clean Up

Everyone loves the smell of fresh, clean laundry. I remember practically huffing my sweaters as a child. I just couldn't get enough of that Snuggle fabric softener scent. Even the Snuggle bear falling into a basket of fluffy blankets during TV commercials made my heart skip a beat. Sure, these products make your laundry smell amazing, but do the benefits outweigh the risks?

Laundry Detergent

Laundry detergents contain an arsenal of chemicals that can make you hormonal and fat, along with a checklist of other health problems. They might take the dirt out but in return they expose you to a throng of chemicals, one being formaldehyde, the toxic chemical used to preserve dead bodies. Some chemicals are known to interfere with hormones, the most common being NPE, or nonylphenol ethoxylate, also known as the "gender bender." Top ingredients to avoid when choosing a laundry detergent include:

- Chlorine bleach (sodium hypochlorite)
- Fragrances (Yes, even lavender oil)
- Phthalates
- Sodium lauryl sulfate (SLS) and sodium laureth sulfate (SLES)
- Brighteners (These ingredients aren't always listed, so a helpful rule of thumb is that if the product is labeled as biodegradable, it probably doesn't contain any brighteners)
- Phosphates & EDTA
- Quaternium-15
- Petroleum distillates
- NPE (nonylphenol ethoxylate)
- Formaldehyde
- 1,4 dioxane

A Note on Borax: Many people who are searching for a chemical-free laundry detergent will be tempted to use borax as an alternative. However, it is a suspected hormone disruptor based on animal studies and it's also toxic to children. It's safest to avoid it.

Non-Toxic Laundry Detergents:

- Seventh Generation laundry detergent, free & clear
- BioKleen free & clear laundry liquid

Fabric Softeners and Dryer Sheets

In-wash fabric softeners and heat-activated dryer sheets pack a powerful combination of chemicals that can harm your health, throw your hormones off balance, damage the environment and pollute the air, both inside and outside your home. I recommend just skipping them completely because there aren't any good options.

Healthy alternatives to fabric softeners and dryer sheets include:

- Distilled white vinegar. Add a half cup to your washing machine during the rinse cycle. The smell doesn't linger on clothes.

- 100% wool dryer balls. They reduce static. You can also reduce static by not over-drying your clothes.

Bleach

Bleach was the first agent of chemical warfare in World War I. Since then, it has been added to our nation's water supply and other products we use at home. The active ingredient in bleach is chlorine, which sabotages your body in a number of ways. It can interfere with estrogen. It can displace iodine, which may result in an underactive thyroid. In addition, studies have even found swimming in chlorinated pools is associated with low testosterone and low sperm quality in boys and men. An unanswered question is, why are we still using it? I literally do not know the answer. There are safer alternatives that you can use to clean or disinfect, including:

- Hydrogen peroxide
- Lemon juice
- Baking soda
- Vinegar
- Citric acid

Non-Toxic Bleach Alternatives:

- Seventh Generation Chlorine-Free Bleach, Free & Clear
- BioKleen Oxygen Bleach Plus

Online Help for Finding Healthy Products

Make your search for cleaner cosmetics, toiletries, and cleaning products easier by checking out Environmental Working Group's consumer guides by visiting ewg.org. They rate personal care products, food, and cleaning products using a score system that shows you how safe a product is, along with healthy living tips. It's a godsend for busy women like me because it saves so much time from researching what I should and shouldn't buy.

PART THREE

Flipping the Menopause Switch

Now that you have had a hormonal primer, you have done the necessary prep work by detoxing your environment, body, and mind, it's time to flip the menopause switch. First, I will introduce you to some very common menopausal symptoms you may be suffering from, then I will recommend specific lifestyle changes you can make to help ease your symptoms. I also included a list of supplements that have been scientifically proven to help, from trusted brands you can count on. If these natural treatments are not enough to relieve your symptoms, then consider hormone replacement therapy.

A note on supplement safety. Taking a supplement can be equivalent to swallowing a pill from a bottle that says, "Eat me," in Alice in Wonderland. It can be dangerous and a waste of your hard-earned money with little to no benefit. Some companies do make high-quality products but there is also a dark world of companies that are dishonest and sell products that do not actually contain what they claim. Since supplements are not approved by the Food and Drug Administration, companies are not required to rigorously test their products. I have done the leg work for you. I know which companies are honest, are of high quality, and send their products out for third party testing. I'll share them with you in each chapter. Also, supplements may interact with certain medications so please consult your physician.

CHAPTER 7
HOT FLASHES

"Wise women don't have hot flashes, they have power surges," — a
book by D. Reid Wallace

If you are a woman in midlife and everyone else around you is wearing a sweater but you're down to a tank top and sweating beads wondering if you're going through menopause, then keep on reading, girlfriend. Hot flashes are one of the hallmarks of menopause. In fact, eight out of 10 American women suffer from hot flashes when they ride the menopause train. They are the most common menopause symptom and "hot flash" is not surprisingly the most frequent search term used in Google.

Women who experience abrupt menopause when their ovaries are surgically removed often suffer severe hot flashes that start right after surgery and typically last longer than those in women who undergo natural menopause. Most women experience hot flashes for 6 months to 2 years, although some studies suggest that the average period is as long as 3 to 5 years. In some women, hot flashes linger for 10 years or more, and older women are known to have occasional hot flashes.

The Start of a Spark

Although their exact cause isn't fully understood, hot flashes are believed to result in changes in the hypothalamus, a small region in the brain that regulates body temperature. It is thought that as hormones fluctuate, the hypothalamus mistakenly senses that a woman is too warm so it signals the body to cool down by enlarging the blood vessels to increase blood flow to the surface of the skin to release body heat. This is why your skin may look red and flushed while having a hot flash. Your skin may also sweat as an attempt to cool down. Some hot flashes are easily tolerated, others are annoying or embarrassing, and others can be debilitating.

During a hot flash, you might have:

- A sudden feeling of warmth radiating through your face and upper body
- Warm skin and perspiration
- Rapid heartbeat
- A flushed appearance with red or pink, blotchy skin
- A chill as the hot flash passes
- Night sweats, this is what happens when you have a hot flash while sleeping

Triggers:

- Stress
- Caffeine
- Alcohol
- Spicy foods
- Heat
- Smoking
- Wearing tight clothing

Hot flashes can also be caused an overactive thyroid and by certain medications including some antidepressants, breast cancer, and osteoporosis drugs. Waking up at night in sweat has also been associated with HIV, tuberculosis, and certain cancers. Your medical provider can rule out these causes.

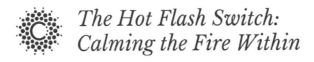

The Hot Flash Switch: Calming the Fire Within

SWITCH #1 Lifestyle Changes

Don't smoke or it will set you on fire. If you don't have enough reasons to quit smoking, here's one more. Smoking may make your hot flashes worse.

Exercise daily. Women who lead a sedentary life seem to suffer more from hot flashes.

Cut back on caffeine. Since the world's most popular drug raises the heart rate, which increases the speed of blood pumping through the body, it can set your internal thermostat even higher and may make hot flashes even worse.

Build your sleep nest. Buy a cooling pillow, fans, cotton sheets, lightweight looser cotton clothing or some women, wearing socks to bed is helpful as it can help to cool core body temperature.

Food remedies. Some research suggests that phytoestrogens, which are plants with estrogen-like effects in the body, can help reduce hot flashes and other menopause symptoms. Examples of plant estrogens include: soybeans, chickpeas, lentils, flaxseed, grains, beans, fruits, red clover and some vegetables. In general, soybeans, chickpeas, and lentils are considered to have the most powerful plant estrogens, though their effect is much less than that of human estrogen.

Deep, paced breathing. When you feel a hot flash coming, take slow, deep breaths to help put yourself into a more relaxed state. You should breathe deeply enough until you feel your diaphragm (the muscular wall beneath your lungs) moving up and down, filling up your lungs completely and then emptying completely. Try taking one deep breath while counting to 4 and then breathe out while counting to 4. You can do this anywhere without anyone knowing so don't worry if you feel silly doing it.

SWITCH #2 Supplements

Black Cohosh is a native North American herb that has a long history of use, originating from Native Americans who used it for treating various ailments and female conditions. Today, it is best known for treating menstrual irregularities and menopausal symptoms including hot flashes and night sweats, vaginal dryness, and moodiness. Studies have found that taking 20-40mg twice a day helps relieve menopausal symptoms by possibly increasing estrogen [27]. There have been some worries that black cohosh is damaging to the liver, however, recent studies suggest that this is very unlikely [28] [29]. You can find this supplement at most natural health stores.

Maca is a native South American plant that has been cultivated as a vegetable for at least 3,000 years. Maca has a very long history of medicinal use. Research has found it to be especially helpful for improving sexual dysfunction in postmenopausal women [30]. I have found that taking 2,000mg per day also helps my female patients struggling with menopausal symptoms. You can also find this supplement at most natural health stores.

St John's Wort. This herb has been used for centuries for the treatment of hot flashes. The recommended dosage is 300mg three times a day. You should consult with your medical provider first before taking this, especially if you are taking an antidepressant, as it may interact with your medications.

Vitamin E is a powerful antioxidant and is recommended for treating menopausal symptoms [31]. Taking 50 to 400IU per day for at least 4 weeks may provide mild relief for hot flashes.

A note on over-the-counter progesterone. There are numerous creams and gels available in stores that contain progesterone. These are often made from wild yams or soybeans and are promoted to help with hot flashes and night sweats. Although they are generally safe and can help some women feel better, the concentrations of hormone and absorption rates can vary greatly. Because of this, they should not be relied upon for uterine protection when taking estrogen.

CHAPTER 8
MOOD SWINGS

"I start each day out as Mary Poppins and end it as Cruella DeVille."
— Author Unknown

I love when a husband tags along for his wife's appointment for a hormone balance consultation. I remember when sweet, quiet Barbara (no last name to protect privacy) came in for the first time. She sat down in my office, alongside her husband, Bill. "I can't take these hot flashes anymore, they're making me miserable." She continued on to tell me about her dry skin, how her hair isn't shiny like it used to be, and that she gained 10 pounds in the past year. I told her that I could help her with these things. That's when Bill chimed in. "Can you make her less crazy, too?" No matter which reproductive phase we are in, premenopause, perimenopause, or menopause, we never get a break from being diagnosed as female crazy. PMS, menopause... Hormone changes can have a significant effect on your mood, but that doesn't mean that you're crazy, it just means that your brain isn't happy with the changes that are happening.

Did You Know?
The word for "uterus" is derived from the Greek root hystera, hence a surgery to remove the uterus is called a "hysterectomy." The root hystera also appears in the words "hysteria" and "hysterical," which, characterized by anxiety, irritability, and ungovernable emotional excess, were historically thought to manifest themselves only in women.

Estrogen helps to regulate several hormones in the brain that are important for mood regulation. These include:

- serotonin
- norepinephrine
- dopamine

Along with falling estrogen levels during midlife come trouble sleeping and issues with sex. Plenty of women also experience anxiety about aging. This menopausal melting pot of body changes, lack of sleep, worry about the future and less enjoyment of sex may contribute to some serious Debbie Downer moments. Although it may seem like you've transitioned into a completely different person, you can start feeling like yourself again with a few tweaks. Aside from managing your hot flashes and night sweats, here are some additional things you can do on your own to turn that frown upside down.

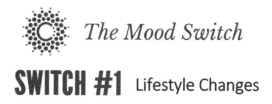 *The Mood Switch*

SWITCH #1 Lifestyle Changes

Carb Brain. Fluctuations in blood sugar can result in rapid mood changes, including low mood and irritability. A diet high in refined carbs like white bread, candy, and soda isn't just bad for your waistline but it can also make you grumpy. Research also suggests it can also lead to depression [32]. Dr. James Gangwisch, a professor at Columbia University, and his team reviewed data of more than 70,000 postmenopausal women from the Women's Health Initiative Study. They found that higher glycemic index scores and eating added sugars and refined grains was associated with a higher risk of depression. The dietary glycemic index, or GI, measures the amount of sugar found in the blood after eating. To give you an idea of how a bagel affects your blood sugar versus broccoli, check out the glycemic index chart below. Basically, the higher the GI number, the more a food spikes your blood sugar.

Glycemic Index

Low GI (<55), Meduim GI (56-69) and High GI (70>)

Grains / Starchs		Vegetables		Fruits		Dairy		Proteins	
Rice Bran	27	Asparagus	15	Grapefruit	25	Low-Fat Yogurt	14	Peanuts	21
Bran Cereal	42	Broccoli	15	Apple	38	Plain Yogurt	14	Beans, Dried	40
Spaghetti	42	Celery	15	Peach	42	Whole Milk	27	Lentils	41
Corn, Sweet	54	Cucumber	15	Orange	44	Soy Milk	30	Kidney Beans	41
Wild Rice	57	Lettuce	15	Grape	46	Fat-Free Milk	32	Split Peas	45
Sweet Potatoes	61	Peppers	15	Banana	54	Skim Milk	32	Lima Beans	46
White Rice	64	Spinach	15	Mango	46	Chocolate Milk	35	Chickpeas	47
Cous Cous	65	Tomatoes	65	Pineapple	66	Fruit Yogurt	36	Pinto Beans	55
Whole Wheat Bread	71	Chickpeas	33	Watermelon	72	Ice Cream	61	Black-Eyed Beans	59
Muesli	80	Cooked Carrots	39						
Baked Potatoes	85								
Oatmeal	87								
Taco Shells	97								
White Bread	100								
Bagel, White	103								

Sugar in small amounts triggers your happiness factor. When you consume sugar, it activates the reward center in the brain, triggering a release of "happy hormones". However, over-activating this reward system kickstarts a series of unfortunate events and if you've ever experienced a sugar crash, then you know that sudden peaks and drops in blood sugar levels can cause your mood to drop along with them. Like I say with everything, stay away from highly refined carbs. It's better for your body and your mind. Fill your plate with mostly vegetables, some proteins, and a little fruit and you'll be a healthier, happier person.

Mind-Body Practices: Tai Chi, Yoga, Qi Gong. It doesn't matter which practice you choose. The purpose of mind-body practices is to help relieve stress and improve sleep, which will ultimately help with your mood.

- **Yoga** is a combination of meditation, controlled breathing, and postures.

- **Qi Gong** is a form of traditional Chinese medicine that combines meditation, breathing, and physical movement.

- **Tai Chi** originated in China and is a series of gentle, flowing movements combined with focused breathing and awareness. It is believed by many to help the qi (chee) flow, meaning vital energy, through the body. Tai chi can be a form of Qi Gong but is generally more complex, more focused on form, and is a martial art whereas Qi Gong is a system of wellness.

Sleep. Not getting enough Zzzz's can bring out the worst in people. It sure does to me! Less than 8 hours and this seemingly pleasant lady turns into the Wicked Witch of the West (my husband can confirm). Check out Chapter 11: Difficulty Sleeping for some solid advice on how to stop counting sheep and start sleeping the recommended 7-8 hours per night.

SWITCH #2 Supplements

Asian Panax Ginseng. There is some evidence that suggests Asian Panax ginseng may help with mood. I recommend starting with 200 mg per day and if that does not help, try 400 mg.

5-HTP. Taking 5-HTP at higher doses, around 200-300mg, has been found to improve depression. I recommend starting with a low dose of 25mg and gradually increasing it until it has an effect. You should never take 5-HTP if you are on antidepressant medication without talking to your doctor first, as this combination can cause serotonin syndrome, a potentially dangerous condition resulting from too much serotonin in the brain.

Rhodiola. This herb has been used for centuries to improve mood. It is suggested that taking 200 mg twice per day improves mood by balancing the neurotransmitters in the brain.

Vitamin D. It's called the "sunshine vitamin" for more than one reason. In addition to bone health, just like the sun, vitamin D has been shown to have a positive effect on low mood. Since mood symptoms are common in the menopause years, anything that minimizes your mood troubles is worth your attention. Many women are deficient in vitamin D, especially after menopause because estrogen increases the activity of an enzyme responsible for activating vitamin D. There are not many foods very rich in vitamin D. Salmon and swordfish are food sources but most people don't get enough vitamin D through diet. Healthy sun exposure is your best bet. You can also take a supplement.

St John's Wort. This herb has been used for centuries for the treatment of depression. The recommended dosage is 300mg three times a day. You should consult with your medical provider first before taking this, especially if you are taking an antidepressant, as it may interact with your medications.

Although adjusting your diet, practicing calming techniques, and supplementing with mood boosters is enough to help many women deal with moodiness resulting from menopause, see a doctor or medical professional if your mood swings are extreme and make it difficult to participate fully in life. Your doctor will want to do a physical exam to rule out any underlying cause for your mood swings and also evaluate you for depression. If symptoms are severe enough, medication might be necessary.

CHAPTER 9

WEIGHT GAIN & SLOWED METABOLISM

"I lied on my Weight Watchers list. I put down that I had 3 eggs... but they were Cadbury chocolate eggs."
— Caroline Rhea

Mirror, mirror, on the wall, who's the biggest witch of all? *The scale.* Brutally honest, there's no way to cheat or lie to this adversary. The numbers on the scale will never fail to remind you of your top-secret midnight date with *Ben & Jerry* and that you traded leg day for a Netflix binge twice last week — when you promised yourself you wouldn't. Ringing any bells?

It's only human to cheat on your diet once in a blue moon... But after your 35th birthday and especially once you hit menopause, you may be doing a lot less "cheating" and a lot more, *"I'm working out, eating right and I can't lose weight – no matter what!"* This can leave you feeling discouraged and frustrated, ready to give up entirely. After all, you want to lose weight not only to look sexy in that bikini and those jeans you've been dying to fit into again but for other benefits like having more energy, looking younger, boosting your sex drive, and lowering your risk of heart disease, diabetes, and cancer. As Dr. Blackburn of Harvard Medical School [33] says, "losing weight is more difficult as we age, but *not impossible.*" So, don't throw in the towel just yet! Truth is, you may be overlooking an uber important part of your biology that could be keeping you from losing weight or causing you to gain weight despite your efforts: your hormones. An imbalance of your hormones as you age causes a perfect storm of fat growth. One where "fat growers" outrank "fat fighters."

Menopausal Muffin Top

As you get older, you might notice that it becomes harder to lose weight and fat seems to prefer gravitating toward your waistline, also known as the dreaded "Menopausal Muffin Top." As fat was once stored in the hips, thighs, and buttocks as a reserve for breastfeeding, it's no longer needed for that purpose when we hit menopause. Most women gain 10 to 15 pounds starting in perimenopause and then a pound a year after that. Thank you, hormones! Fat moves to the abdominal area instead and becomes toxic visceral (deep belly) fat, which can cause inflammation in the body and can increase risk of diabetes, heart disease, and cancer. As a general rule, if your waist is greater than 35 inches around, you have too much "toxic" belly fat. Your body mass index can also be a good indicator. Check out appendix A in the back of this book for a Body Mass Index (BMI) chart.

The Stress Connection

Stress causes cortisol levels to rise, and if this occurs over a prolonged period of time, you can develop food cravings and blood sugar imbalances, leading to fat storage. Cortisol, also known as the "stress hormone," is produced in the adrenal glands and helps regulate glucose (blood sugar) levels and metabolism. Similarly, it is insulin's job to tell the cells in your body how to use glucose. Your body can either use glucose as energy or store it as fat. So, when it comes to stress and weight gain, the problem is twofold: When you experience a lot of stress, your cortisol levels rise, which makes your body less sensitive to insulin and therefore your cells aren't able to use it for energy and it is then stored as fat. In addition, a high cortisol level from stress makes you crave sugar, so you're more likely to eat high-carbohydrate meals, which spike your blood sugar and your insulin level, which further contributes to fat storage. It's a vicious cycle: You're stressed, cortisol levels rise, you become tired and hungry, you eat a high-carb diet because of it, which raises your blood sugar level, which raises your insulin level, which contributes to insulin resistance and fat storage.

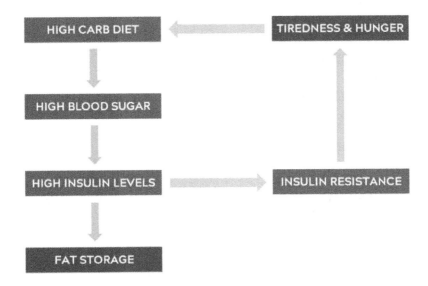

In addition, insulin resistance can occur if your blood sugar and insulin levels remain high for a long time. Your cells have a difficult time taking in the glucose to use it as fuel, so it begins to build up in your bloodstream. Since your cells are having such a hard time using that energy, they starve and send out stress signals. This is where cortisol comes in to play again. Cortisol is a hormone that responds to stress, which causes fat storage. Also, any extra sugar that isn't used and is floating around in your blood is sent to the liver to be store as glycogen for use at a later time, and if there is too much, it is stored as fat.

When Supply Outperforms Demand

Remember, our metabolism slows down as we age which means that it's harder to burn off calories. Unfortunately, even though we don't need as many calories as we did in our 20's, we will still want to eat and drink the same amount as before. The average calorie needs for women during lifespan are:

<u>Sedentary</u>
19 to 25- 2,000 calories
26 to 50- 1,800 calories
Age 50 and up- 1,600 calories

<u>Moderately Active</u>
19 to 25- 2,200 calories
26 to 50- 2,000 calories
Age 50 and up- 1,800 calories

<u>Very Active</u>
19 to 30- 3,000 calories
31 to 60- 2,200 calories
Age 61 and up- 2,000 calories

Since it takes 3,500 extra calories to gain one pound of fat, just adding an extra muffin (approximately 500 calories) to your breakfast each morning can cause you to gain a pound a week! Unless you exercised it off, but that means you would have to run around 6 miles a day (approximately 500 calories) to burn off those morning muffins. That would also mean that you need to have the energy to run 6 miles a day and it's a bit hard to do so when you may be tired because you aren't sleeping well and are woken up by hot flashes, your husband wanting to make love to you when your vagina is as dry as the desert and you have to get up to pee every few hours.

The Secret to Weight Loss

The secret to weight loss is really simple: Eat less calories than you burn. If you consistently burn all of the calories that you consume in the course of a day, you will maintain your weight. If you consume more energy (calories) than you burn, you will gain weight. That doesn't mean simple is easy though. There are many other factors that make weight loss seem nearly impossible. Hunger, cravings, and health problems can make it hard to eat the right foods in the right amounts, pushing the numbers on the scale in the opposite direction than you want.

Calories are Complex

Counting calories is complicated and time-consuming and if you are getting most of your calories from the wrong foods, your body will respond by shifting your hormones and triggering your brain to want to eat more than you really need. Although a calorie is a calorie (a unit of energy), not all calories are created equal when it comes to your health because different foods have different effects on various processes in your body. For example, 500 calories worth of chicken breast will have a very different effect on your body than 500 calories of white bread. Eating the chicken would help you feel satisfied longer because of the protein, while the white bread would satisfy you only for a short period of time, leading to eating more and consuming too many calories.

Low-Fat versus Low-Carb

Dietary fat doesn't necessarily make you fat. In fact, the excessive amount of refined carbohydrates (bread, pasta, pastries) and sugar in the typical American diet is arguably to blame. In 1977, the United States government made its very first dietary recommendation to "eat less fat and cholesterol, and more carbohydrates" [34]. The obesity rate in America thus skyrocketed and the rate of diabetes went up along with it. The recommendation was a big fat fail (literally). Americans consumed more refined carbohydrates (do you remember Wonder Bread?) along with less fiber, which not only contributed to us as a nation getting fatter, but also more likely to develop type 2 diabetes [35].

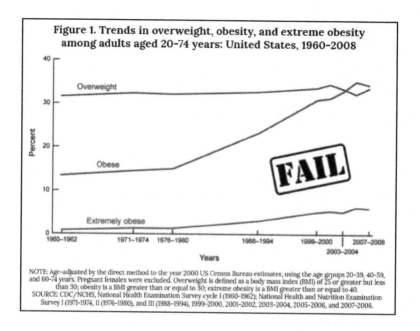

Figure 1. Trends in overweight, obesity, and extreme obesity among adults aged 20-74 years: United States, 1960-2008

NOTE: Age-adjusted by the direct method to the year 2000 US Census Bureau estimates, using the age grpups 20-39, 40-59, and 60-74 years. Pregnant females were excluded. Overweight is defined as a body mass index (BMI) of 25 or greater but less than 30; obesity is a BMI greater than or equal to 30; extreme obesity is a BMI greater than or equal to 40.
SOURCE: CDC/NCHS, National Health Examination Survey cycle I (1960-1962); National Health and Nutrition Examination Survey I (1971-1974), II (1976-1980), and III (1988-1994), 1999-2000, 2001-2002, 2003-2004, 2005-2006, and 2007-2008.

Fat is essential in our diet and we need it to build and maintain many parts of our body including our hormones. Research suggests that a low-carbohydrate, higher fat diet can significantly reduce body weight [36]. Diets high in healthy fats (such as keto) tend to be very filling because the higher amount of fats sends a signal to the brain that the body has taken in enough energy (calories) to be used. Since the focus is on healthy fats and whole foods, you actually may reduce overeating of empty calories and junk food. So, the next time you are at the grocery store, avoid the "reduced fat" foods and choose foods that are in their natural state.

Reasons to NOT buy low-fat foods include:

- Eating fat makes you feel satisfied. When you eat fat, your brain receives signals that you have the needed energy stores coming in and your appetite is then suppressed. Your stomach starts to empty more slowly, which means that you end up feeling full longer. Low-fat foods don't have the same effect. You end up eating more calories because your body doesn't sense that enough energy is coming in.

- Displacing carbs with fat helps with weight loss because of the effect on insulin. Insulin is a hormone that is released by your pancreas in proportion to the amount of carbs you eat. The more carbs you eat, the more insulin is released. But the more insulin released, the more weight gain. Keeping insulin levels low helps you lose weight. Fat in the diet helps keep insulin levels low and allows your body to use fat as energy.

- When you get enough fat in your diet, your body becomes conditioned to burn it more efficiently. This has to do with a fat-burning hormone called adiponectin, which is produced when you eat fat. Adiponectin increases the rate that fats are broken down, curbs appetite, increases muscle efficiency, and increases insulin sensitivity. When you eat low-fat foods, only small amounts of adiponectin are produced. You want to keep those numbers high.

Worried about cholesterol? Cholesterol in food only has a small effect on the level of cholesterol in your blood [37]. It just so turns out that the amount of calories from fat is irrelevant and replacing fat with refined carbs and sugar is far worse. Do you remember the good ole American slogan: "The incredible, edible egg?" Chicken eggs are high in cholesterol, but the effect of egg consumption on blood cholesterol is minimal. The risk of heart disease may be more closely tied to the foods that accompany the eggs in a traditional American breakfast.

Did You Know?
Eggs are the ONLY food that contain ALL the essential amino acids? Amino acids are the building blocks of proteins and are also responsible for the productions of hormones. It's no wonder the saying goes, "The incredible, edible egg."

You should strive for a balance of healthy fats, protein, and complex carbohydrates during every meal. The keyword for carbs is "complex." This means you should be including fresh fruits and vegetables and whole grains in your diet to cover the carbohydrate portion, while avoiding or minimizing refined carbs such as white bread, pasta, and pastries.

Good Fats & Bad Fats

A general rule of thumb is that "good fats" come from whole foods. That includes fruit and vegetables, nuts and seeds, fish, eggs... You get the idea. "Good fats" from whole foods, such as olive oil, have positive effects on your body and support healthy hormone balance. "Bad fats" that have been highly processed, such as hydrogenated oils, throw off your hormone balance by blocking the actions of "good fats."

Good Fats and Bad Fats

Good Fats		OK But Not Great	Bad Fats	
Traditionally used Fats and Oils		Refined Traditional Fats	Polyunsaturated	Trans
Not Highly processed, and not refined		Label says 'Refined'	Refined Bleached Deodorized	Label says 'Hydrogenated'
All Purpose	Caution w/ Heat	Limited Use	Don't Eat	
Olive Oil	Walnut Oil	Refined Peanut	Soy Oil	Fake whip cream
Avocado Oil	Flax Oil	Refined Avocado	Sunflower Oil	Fake butter spreads
Peanut Oil	Sesame	Refined Coconut	Safflower Oil	Store-bought pastries
Butter/Ghee	Walnuts		Canola Oil	Chicken Nuggets
Tallow & Lard	Seeds		Corn Oil	Margarine
Cocoa Butter	Fatty Fish		Cottonseed Oil	Shortening
Mac Nut Oil	Artisanal Grapeseed		Hydrogenated Oil	Restaurant fried foods
Coconut Oil			Refined Palm	Most chips & crackers
Almond Oil				Most protien bars
Unrefined Palm			Mostly in Restaurants:	Most salad dressings
Palm Kernel Oil			Grapeseed Oil	Most mayo brands
			Ricebran Oil	Most granola & cereal

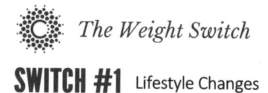

The Weight Switch

SWITCH #1 Lifestyle Changes

Weigh yourself every week. Some people may dispute that, arguing that it's unhealthy to obsess over numbers on the scale but in my opinion (take this advice from someone who has lost over 50 pounds), knowing what the numbers are will help you pay more attention to what you eat. If you gained 2 pounds over the weekend, you'll probably be more mindful when your coworkers bring in a box full of bagels on Monday morning. Vice versa, if you have been working on your diet and staying more active and you see the numbers on the scale go down, you'll feel motivated to keep on going. If you weigh yourself daily, keep in mind that daily variations may be caused by hormones that affect fluid retention.

Join the Sugar-Free Revolution. Listen closely because this is probably the best weight loss advice I am going to tell you: Sugar is the main reason your old jeans haven't been worn for years. Sugar is thy enemy. It's addictive, it's found in abundance, and it will kill you after it makes you fat, crabby, and depressed.

Did You Know?
Research has found that people who consume large quantities of artificial sweeteners gain more weight, not lose it. This may be due to how the gut flora (bacteria and other microbes living in your intestinal tract) respond to the chemicals in it. Just put that pink packet down. I think most of us can agree it tastes terrible anyway.

Break Away from the Box. This is the second most important weight loss advice I am going to give you: If it doesn't look like it grew from the ground, don't put it in your mouth. Macaroni and cheese didn't grow from the ground. It's not natural to eat it. Healthy foods don't usually come in boxes nor are they included in "buy one, get one free sales." I also want to warn you about commercial "weight loss systems" that involve packaged meals that are delivered to your door. Be wary if the meals consist of hamburgers, pizza, and pasta, even though they are low-calorie. This is not learning how to make better food choices and once you go off their diet, you'll be right back where you were before, ordering a Big Mac at McDonald's and the vicious weight gain comes back full speed. That's why these companies make so much money, because it's simply a yo-yo diet where people are taught to continue buying processed foods that are high in refined carbohydrates. Not to mention, these foods aren't nutritionally dense. You need to learn to eat whole food, not factory food.

The Big "O." Not the toe-curling kind (although that exercise is a great way to get your cardio in). What I mean is organic. Choose organic foods as much as possible. Many beef cattle raised on conventional farms are injected with hormones to fatten them up, which is still in the meat when it ends up on your plate. Chickens are often given antibiotics to help them survive horrid, disease-laden living conditions, which are still in the meat and eggs that they produce. Conventionally farmed fruits and vegetables are sprayed with pesticides and grown in soil fertilized with poisonous chemicals. Organic foods may cost a little more but by eating organic, you are investing in your health by reducing your exposure to toxic pesticides, fertilizers, and hormones that can interfere with your own hormone balance.

A note on buying organic: If you absolutely cannot buy all of your food organic, at least make sure that the animal products are, as toxins are concentrated in fatty tissue, which means you're getting a far more potent dose of toxic chemicals with animal products than with fruits and vegetables.

Lift. As testosterone levels decline through midlife, muscle mass decreases and it leaves you feeling weak and flabby. Less muscle means lower metabolism and weight gain. One of the secrets of fitness for older women is lifting weights. Building muscle will help you burn more calories. Cardio exercise such as walking and biking is great for your heart and does burn calories, but adding on weight lifting to your exercise routine will get you closer to your weight loss goals in less time. Lifting weights is also a great way to lower your chances of developing osteoporosis, which commonly affects women after menopause. Don't go into it blindly though because you can hurt yourself if you don't know what you're doing. Most gyms offer a free introductory lesson with a personal trainer so take advantage of it so you can use the equipment properly and stay safe.

Go Non-GMO. While you are shopping around in the grocery store, here's something to think about: More than 75% of the processed foods on those shelves are made from genetically modified organisms (GMOs). GMOs are living organisms whose genetic material has been artificially manipulated in a laboratory through genetic engineering to do things they don't naturally do: Withstand the application of herbicides, produce insecticides, or even resist browning in apples. They are the Frankensteins of our refrigerators and this is a recent lab experiment we are doing with food, which means there's not enough research to prove their safety for human consumption. The first ever commercially grown GMO product to be approved for consumption was a tomato in 1994. Now, if we fast forward to today, the list of GMO products is longer than ever. The top 10 most common GMO foods include:

- Alfalfa
- Aspartame (artificial sweetener made from genetically modified bacteria)
- Animal products
- Canola
- Corn
- Papaya
- Potato
- Soy
- Sugar beet
- Summer squash/zucchini

Scary Fact: More than 80% of all GMO crops worldwide have been engineered to withstand herbicide. As a result, the use of toxic herbicides, such as Roundup®, has increased fifteenfold. In March 2015, the World Health Organization determined that the herbicide glyphosate (the key ingredient in Roundup®) is "probably" carcinogenic to humans. Just imagine how many would be harmed before "probably" changes to "definitely."

You might be wondering, what do GMOs have to do with my hormone health? The answer is that we really don't know. Since GMO products are still new to human consumption, there isn't enough research to truly know the long-term effects on health.

Not all food manufacturers are required to disclose their products are GMO. So, while you are shopping for groceries look for products, choose organic first. The use of GMOs is prohibited in organic products. If you do not buy an organic product, look for a "non-GMO" label. These companies, although not organic, take pride in not using GMOs.

SWITCH #2 Supplements

You have no idea how many people walk into my clinic hoping to take a magical pill to lose weight. I am the deliverer of bad news: You have to put in the work to reap the benefit.

Changing your diet is the #1 way to lose weight. Exercise is #2. Stress management is #3. Supplements are at the trail end at #4 but only with minimal to modest effects. Let me also warn you that the weight loss industry is a cash cow, worth $72 billion in 2018 [38] and because it's a business and in it to make money, it relies on people losing weight, gaining the weight back, losing it again, and so on. Repeat business means a constant cash flow. People will spend a lot of money to lose weight and feel better about themselves and that's part of the reason why the weight loss industry is so successful, aside from the fact modern Americans have almost forgotten what healthy food is. There are a ton of supplements on store shelves promising weight loss. I am going to list only the supplements that have been proven by a decent amount of research to help people lose weight.

Fiber. Women should consume 35 to 45 grams per day or more. Considering the average American adult only eats 15 grams of fiber per day, I recommend supplementation. Psyllium seed husk is a great fiber supplement that contains 70% soluble fiber, which means it can help increase fullness and slow digestion. You can also buy it anywhere. Make sure you drink plenty of water with it because it absorbs loads of water.

Conjugated linoleic acid (CLA) is found primarily in beef and dairy products, so if you're vegetarian or vegan, you likely aren't getting enough. This powerful antioxidant reduces body fat while preserving muscle. In addition, it helps lower cholesterol, triglycerides, and blood pressure. The best way to get CLA is through diet but supplements are also available and effective. Taking up to 3 grams per day seems safe.

Capsaicin. Naturally spicy (plus anti-inflammatory) ingredients like cayenne, black pepper, turmeric, ginger, or cinnamon might help increase your body's ability to burn fat, suppress hunger levels, normalize glucose levels, reduce free radical damage associated with aging and reduce your appetite for sweets. Capsaicin, the phytochemical responsible for the spiciness of peppers, has been shown to speed up metabolism [39], so try spicing up to slim down.

Acetyl-L-carnitine is an amino acid naturally produced in your body to generate energy. It's also found in red meat. It helps your mitochondria (the powerhouses of your cells) burn fat and create more energy. Take 1 gram 90 minutes before exercise to increase muscle endurance and 1 gram after exercise (to speed up recovery).

Green coffee bean extract comes from coffee beans that haven't been roasted. Coffee beans contain compounds known as chlorogenic acids. Some believe these compounds have antioxidant effects, help lower blood pressure, and help you lose weight. Roasting coffee reduces chlorogenic acid content. This is why drinking coffee isn't thought to have the same weight loss effects as the unroasted beans. The extract is sold as a pill and can be found online or in health food stores, with typical doses between 60 to 185 mg per day.

Green Tea Extract is an amazing energy and metabolism booster. When green tea extract is produced, catechins (antioxidant compounds) called "ECGC" are isolated from the plant and are used in high concentrations. These have powerful effects and can act as appetite suppressants.

Green tea extract can also help mobilize fat from fat cells for use as energy, by inhibiting fat-burning hormones in the body. A study published in the American Journal of Clinical Nutrition [40] found that consuming green tea before exercise has been shown to burn 17% more fat. It seems safe for most adults to take up to 800–900 milligrams daily, usually spread out over three increments [41].

CHAPTER 10
BRAIN FOG

"My mind is like my internet browser. Nineteen tabs are open, three of them are frozen, and I have no idea where the music is coming from." — *Author unknown*

How many times have you been in a situation when you're having a conversation with someone and you say something like, "That reminds me of a movie I saw once with that blonde actress, you know, the one when she falls in love with Matthew McConaughey...Hmm... She was also in that movie *Legally Blonde*. Gosh, it's at the tip of my tongue..?" It's like the name is right there but you can't bring it down from your brain to your lips. If you have also found yourself more frequently walking into the kitchen to get something and it takes a few minutes to figure out what it was by the time you got there, you may be suffering from "Meno-fog." Finding it hard to concentrate and taking longer than usual to remember things does not always mean that you have dementia. It could just mean that your menopausal brain is making it harder for you to function at your highest cognitive capacity.

Fluctuating levels of estrogen during perimenopause and falling levels during menopause can make it difficult for your brain's estrogen receptors to meet their requirements, causing brain fog, forgetfulness, and a lack of focus. Our brain also ages, which means that the most important parts involved with higher cognitive function, such as the frontal lobe and hippocampus, shrink. We also slow down production of important neurotransmitters (chemical messengers) and lose some of their connection points. In addition, the protective coating of our nerve fibers (myelin sheath) deteriorates, slowing down brain processes.

This may all sound scary to you but don't fret. This does not mean that you are developing dementia. In fact, the typical brain fog associated with perimenopause and menopause come nowhere close to the severe and debilitating effects of dementia. Taking a few minutes to remember a name or why you went to the kitchen to get something is very common around the time of menopause. Not remembering your own name or how to get home is something more serious. Alzheimer's disease, the most common form of dementia, usually affects women older than 65, more so in the 80's. Although our modern advances in medicine can help medical professionals diagnose Alzheimer's disease earlier than ever, the only way to actually confirm its diagnosis is by performing an autopsy. An autopsy of the brain will show amyloid plaques and neurofibrillary tangles, which are characteristic of Alzheimer's disease.

Risk Factors for Alzheimer's Disease

- Older age (65 years or older)
- Family history of Alzheimer's disease, as there is a genetic link
- Diabetes
- High blood pressure
- High cholesterol
- History of stroke
- History of repeated head injuries

 The Brain Fog Switch: Combat Menopause Brain and Protect Yourself from Dementia

SWITCH #1 Lifestyle Changes

Exercise regularly. The best scientific evidence out there for boosting brain activity and preventing dementia is regular cardio exercise, also known as aerobic exercise. This means exercising at a moderate level of intensity over a long period of time, which increases your breathing and heart rate. This allows your body to use the maximum amount of oxygen and a highly oxygenated brain means a better functioning brain. It can also keep your heart, lungs, and circulatory system healthy. Examples of aerobic exercise include brisk walking, jogging, running, cycling, and swimming.

Socialize. Maintaining a social network is beneficial to your brain health. As you may know, social interaction is a key to brain development during childhood. However, it is also important as you age since it can help prevent and also slow down mental decline. In fact, social interaction has been linked to a lower risk of dementia including Alzheimer's disease. An extensive research study [42] explored the role of social activity among people with dementia. Researchers from John Hopkins and Duke University assessed 147 pairs of male twins over an average of 28 years, following them for signs and predictors of dementia. The results showed that participants with greater leisurely cognitive activity in their midlife, including social engagement, experienced a significant delay in the onset of dementia. In fact, social activities such as visiting relatives and friends, participating in a club and attending parties were most strongly linked to a lower risk of dementia, as were cognitive tasks like studying and reading. With that in mind, activities that combine social engagement with cognitive function may provide the best protection against Alzheimer's, according to the study.

Unfortunately, aging adults often find themselves becoming more isolated as they get older. Five ways to remain socially engaged at an older age include:

- Joining a senior activity center. Most centers offer free or at least very affordable activities that make it easy to connect with other people in the same stage of life. Shy? Hesitant to go by yourself? Keep in mind that everyone else is there for the exact same reason you are: to have a good time, create and maintain friendships, and keep active.
- Joining a game club. One of the best ways to make new social contacts and keep your mind sharp is to play games. Regardless of your interests, skill level or physical ability, there's a game out there to suit your needs: Crossword puzzles, bridge, Sudoku (number puzzles), chess, and nearly every other game out there. Don't worry if you're not experienced. Veteran game players love showing their skills to

newbies. Soon enough you'll be teaching some other newbie the tricks of the game.

- Volunteering. Helping out in the community is not only a great way to feel good about the good deeds you are doing, but it's also a great way to socialize. The opportunities to volunteer are endless. Pick something you think you would enjoy doing. Love animals? Offer to help out at your local Humane Society or SPCA. Love kids? Get involved with a local literacy program that works to improve kids' reading levels. There are also "foster grandparent" programs in which you can work directly as a friend and positive role model for at-risk youth. Other great places to volunteer include the local library, hospital, and community soup kitchen.

Mindfulness-Based Stress Reduction (MBSR). High levels of chronic stress can negatively impact your brain. Practicing MBSR can help combat the effects of chronic stress, which may improve brain function. When I was working on a research study [43] on the effects of MBSR on breast cancer survivors, we found that it did help women who were suffering from "chemo brain," thinking and memory problems that can occur during and after cancer treatment. Additional research has also found that practicing MBSR is associated with an increase in gray matter in brain regions involved in learning and memory processes [44].

SWITCH #2 Supplements

Nootropics are natural supplements or drugs that have a beneficial effect on brain function in healthy people. Many of these can boost memory, motivation, creativity, alertness and general cognitive function and may also reduce age-related declines in brain function. Some examples of nootropics include:

Acetyl-L-carnitine is an amino acid found naturally in your body and has been found that taking 1,500 to 3,000 mg per day may slow down age-related decline in brain function and improve memory in people with dementia.

Fish oil supplements are a rich source of docosahexaenoic acid (DHA) and eicosapentaenoic acid (EPA), two types of omega-3 fatty acids that are backed by science to improve brain health [45]. DHA plays a vital role in maintaining the structure and function of your brain and EPA has an anti-inflammatory effect which may protect your brain against aging. Overall, the best way to get the recommended amount of omega-3 fatty acids is by eating two 3.5 ounce portions of fatty fish (i.e. salmon, albacore tuna) per week, however, most people don't and that's when taking a supplement can be beneficial. Taking 1 gram a day (equal to 1,000 mg) of fish oil containing EPA and DHA is generally recommended to maintain brain health

Gingko Biloba: Traditional Chinese medicine has used the fan-shaped leaves of the gingko tree to treat all kinds of ailments. The extract from the leaves of the gingko tree is sold as a supplement known as ginkgo biloba. Some research suggests that it improves memory in older adults by improving blood flow to the brain [46] [47]. Taking 120mg per day may help support your memory and reduce brain fog.

Phosphatidylserine is a type of fat compound called a phospholipid and since it is found in your brain, taking 300mg per day may help preserve your brain and reduce age-related decline in brain function and improve memory [48].

Resveratrol is an antioxidant found in the skin of red and purple fruits such as grapes and blueberries. For your reading pleasure, get this: red wine is a source of resveratrol. But I don't recommend you start an alcohol habit thinking it will benefit your brain. One glass of red wine only contains 0.2 to 2 mg of resveratrol and although there have not been a lot of studies on its effects on brain health, one study suggested that taking 200mg of resveratrol per day improved memory in older adults [49]. That would mean you'd have to drink about 100 glasses of wine to get as much resveratrol as you would from a capsule. Since only drinking moderately (1 glass per day for women, 2 glasses per day for men) has been associated with good health, any more than that actually reverses its benefits.

Vitamins B6, B9, and B12 help protect the brain by breaking down homocysteine, an amino acid in your blood which in high levels have been associated with an increased risk of dementia and Alzheimer's disease. These important vitamins are also necessary for the development of new brain cells. Meat is the highest food source of B vitamins. Most people get enough B vitamins through their diet, however, those who do not eat meat, are elderly, and those who take certain medications such as acid blockers may not get enough through diet. Taking a vitamin B complex may help.

Vitamin E is believed to help brain health by reducing oxidative stress. A less than optimal intake of vitamin E has been associated with cognitive decline. Unfortunately, 90% of the American population does not consume the recommended daily allowance of 15 mg/day but average closer to half that value—around 7 mg/day [50]. Foods high in vitamin E include sunflower seeds, almonds, spinach, and avocadoes. Additionally, taking a supplement up to 1,000mg (1,500 IU) per day is considered safe for most adults.

CHAPTER 11
DIFFICULTY SLEEPING

"My bed is a magical place where I suddenly remember everything I was supposed to do." — Author unknown

Sleeping difficulties are the second most common complaint of women going through menopause. Considering we spend a third of our lives sleeping, it shouldn't be a waste of our precious time. For anyone who knows me, I'm strict when it comes to my sleep schedule. In my opinion, there's nothing worse than a bad night's sleep because no matter how much you think you can conquer the next day, after spending hours tossing and turning in bed, you will not have the ability to think as clearly, stay on task, or make good choices as you would if you had gotten 8 hours of high-quality sleep. Not to mention, there are health consequences that follow, including an increased risk for high blood pressure, heart disease, diabetes, and depression.

If you have difficulty falling asleep, wake up in the middle of the night, or wake too early in the morning, you are not alone. According to the National Sleep Foundation [51], almost 50% of American women age 40 and older are having the same problems you are. Not coincidentally, other studies have indicated that the closer women get to menopause, the more sleep trouble. As hormone levels fall, their interactions with special brain chemicals (neurotransmitters) that help us sleep fall as well, which makes it harder to fall and stay asleep.

Other Sleep Vampires

Hot flashes, night sweats, and having to pee are common sleep vampires for women going through menopause. There are other conditions that are common during midlife that will keep you counting sheep until the cows come home. These may include:

- Restless legs syndrome
- Sleep apnea
- Depression/Anxiety
- Chronic pain
- Chronic health issues
- Nighttime urinary frequency
- Certain medications

In addition, stress from life circumstances can also interfere with your ability to sleep. This may include:

- Divorce
- Death of a friend or family member
- Loss of job or recent retirement
- Relocation to a new home
- Children moving away
- Caregiving for elderly parents
- Change in routine such as less exercise

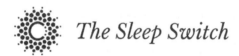 *The Sleep Switch*

So how can you flip the switch on sleep? How can you turn the brain volume down and the ZZZ's back up? First, let's start with healthy sleep habits and then I will reveal what therapies may help. I always recommend exhausting all natural options first before surrendering to prescription medications, as these can not only be habit-forming but they can also leave you feeling groggy the next day.

SWITCH #1 Lifestyle Changes

Stick to a schedule. Go to bed around the same time every night and wake up around the same time every morning, regardless if you work or not. A consistent pattern may be exactly what you need.

Relax before bed. Create a ritual that can help you prepare for sleep. Whether it's taking a warm bath or reading a book, choose something that you enjoy and calms you down as long as it doesn't involve screens. Cellphones, TVs, and computers emit blue light that can interfere with your sleep-wake cycle and prevent you from falling asleep. Remember that your bedroom is only for sleep and sex.

Leave your worries on the nightstand. If you're a nighttime worrier, clear your head by keeping a notebook on your nightstand and empty your thoughts onto paper before you shut off the lights. Don't want to forget something in the morning? Write it down. It will be there in the morning.

Ban Blue Light. The blue light that's emitted from your cell phone, laptop, tablet, TV, and other screens can delay the release of melatonin, a sleep-inducing hormone that increases alertness and resets the body's internal clock (or circadian rhythm) to a later schedule. Light from fluorescent bulbs and LED lights can also produce the same effect. You should break away from blue light 1-2 hours before bedtime or install an app that automatically warms up the colors on the screen—away from blues and toward reds and yellows—at sunset.

Avoid or limit caffeine and alcohol. The glass of wine before bed might sound like a great way to wind down but although alcohol might help you fall asleep, it actually prevents you from getting enough deep sleep and may cause you to wake up in the middle of the night. Avoid caffeine after lunch, which isn't only in coffee, tea, soda and energy drinks (please tell me you don't drink those) but is also found in chocolate. Sadly for you nighttime chocolate cravers, there is just as much caffeine in a 30 gram piece of dark chocolate as in a 30ml shot of espresso.

Get the Early Bird Special. Eating too much late in the evening can upset your stomach and cause digestion issues that keep you awake, so either eat dinner earlier or keep your bedtime snack small. Also, don't drink too much before bed or you'll wake up to use the bathroom during the night.

Exercise daily and only during the day. Get at least 30 minutes of exercise every day but do it earlier in the day, at least 5-6 hours before bedtime. Activity during the day can help you sleep better at night but exercising too close to your bedtime can keep you awake. **Cigarettes: no ifs, ands, or butts.** Nicotine is a stimulant, which means it can keep you awake if you smoke frequently or close to bedtime. It can also alter the expression of clock genes in your brain, which affects your body's sleep/wake cycle [52]. People who smoke are also 2.5 times more likely to suffer from obstructive sleep apnea, a potentially serious sleep disorder [53].

Mindfulness-Based Stress Reduction (MBSR). In the 1970's, Dr. Jon Kabat-Zinn promoted MBSR, a stress reduction program based on ancient Buddhist principles. MBSR uses mindfulness meditation, body awareness, and yoga to promote awareness of the present moment and it has been shown to lower cortisol [54] and improve sleep. In fact, when I was working at the University of South Florida on a multi-million dollar study, *MBSR Symptom Cluster Trial for Breast Cancer Survivors*, we found that the women who were enrolled in our MBSR class slept longer and didn't wake up as much as those who were not [55]. MBSR is very helpful if it is difficult for you to quiet your mind during moments of rest and sleep. There are plenty of MBSR classes out there and if you can't find one in your neighborhood, there are online options too.

Simple 5 Minute Meditation

- **Make the time.** Set aside just 5 minutes to practice meditation before bed. Set a quiet tone on your phone or an egg timer to keep track of time.

- **Embrace your place.** You don't need a special place to meditate. Anywhere in your house is fine as long as you will be uninterrupted.
- **Get comfortable.** You can sit, lie down, stand, or walk.

- **Breathe deeply.** Focus yourself by breathing deeply and slowly and listen to the air entering and leaving your body. If you start paying attention to other noises around you, such as a fan, refocus on the sounds of your breathing and let the background noise drain out.

- **Focus on your body.** Pay attention to how you feel, scanning your body from your scalp all the way to the tips of your toes. Notice the areas that are relaxed or tense.

- **Reflect.** Once the 5-minute timer goes off, take a deep breath and think about how you feel. Are you more relaxed? Do you feel more centered?

SWITCH #2 Supplements

Cannabidiol (CBD) is a compound found in cannabis that has recently been in the research spotlight for treating a wide array of disorders. Although CBD does not trigger a "high," it has been found to have a calming effect and research suggests taking 160 to 300mg in the evening is an effective treatment for anxiety and sleep disorders [56] [57].

Kava Kava is a member of the nightshade family of plants and is native to the South Pacific islands. It has been used by Pacific islanders as a ceremonial drink to promote relaxation. Research has found 250mg of Kava per day was effective at lowering anxiety which leads to better sleep.
Lavender is a flowering plant widely known for its pleasing scent and sedating effects. Research has found that taking 80mg is effective at lowering anxiety [58].

L-theanine is an amino acid found in green tea that is proven effective at lowering stress-related symptoms such as sleeping difficulties as well as brain function. Taking 200mg before bedtime may promote relaxation to help you fall asleep [59].

Magnesium is a mineral that is important for muscle and nerve health. It can help with occasional sleep difficulties by promoting a sense of calm. Magnesium also has a laxative effect so do not take high doses as it can cause diarrhea, nausea, and abdominal cramping. There are many forms of magnesium. Magnesium glycinate is less likely to cause these effects. A common dosage for sleep is 400mg taken at bedtime. However, talk to your doctor before taking a dose higher than 350mg per day or if you have been prescribed a low-magnesium diet.

Melatonin is a hormone that regulates the sleep-wake cycle. It is made by the pineal gland in the brain but is also available as an over-the-counter supplement. Taking 1mg to 3mg two hours before bedtime has been proven effective for treating sleep disorders. I find that taking a time-release melatonin tablet can help you stay asleep longer than regular.

Valerian root is often referred to as "nature's Valium." It is an herb that has been used since ancient times to promote a sense of calm and improve sleep. Studies suggest that taking 300 to 900mg per day, 30 minutes to 2 hours before bedtime, may help you fall asleep, stay asleep, and have higher quality sleep [60].

5-Hydroxytryptophan (5-HTP) is a compound made naturally in the body and is also sold as a supplement make from the seeds of a plant, Griffonia simplicfolia, which is native to West Africa.
It helps the body produce more serotonin and melatonin, our happy brain chemicals involved in sleep and mood. Taking 5-HTP may help your ability to feel good during the day and sleep restfully at night. It may also help with appetite control and menopausal symptoms. However, lower doses starting at 25mg may improve sleep. I recommend starting with the lowest effective dose of 25mg and gradually increasing it until it has an effect. Talk with your doctor before taking this supplement as it may interfere with certain medications such as antidepressants.

CHAPTER 12

SEXUAL PROBLEMS

"The only time a woman has a true orgasm is when she's shopping." — Joan Rivers

If you'd rather be doing laundry than having sex, then keep on reading. Menopause means you are no longer able to make babies. But that doesn't mean you want to stop practicing. Your vagina might be saying no but your mind might be saying yes. Or maybe it's the other way around. Regardless, if you are suffering from any of these symptoms, you're not alone:

- Vaginal dryness
- Pain during sex
- Low sexual desire
- Low sexual arousal
- Difficulty reaching orgasm

The transition to menopause brings changes to your sex drive, your vagina, and your sexual confidence. Luckily, there are plenty of tricks to help restore your sex life and keep you feeling like the sexy lady you are meant to be. Every woman deserves to feel attractive, seductive, and spicy, no matter what their age is or if they are in a relationship or not. First, let's look at what happens to our lady parts as we transition through menopause, why we suffer from sexual changes, and what can be done about it.

The Bust in Lust

It's a normal process for your sex drive to fluctuate. It's common for your sex life to be revved up at the beginning of a relationship but damper down as you enter into a more restful phase with your partner in later years. It's also common to feel like a cat in heat until you have a baby that wakes you up at 12am, 3am, and 6am. Life circumstances happen and can change things. But hormones can change things too. Sexual desire relies on hormones and it can fizz out as hormone levels drop during menopause. As estrogen and testosterone levels fall, our brains aren't as sexually stimulated as they used to be. Physical changes in your body can lower your sexual desire, too. Vaginal dryness leads to painful sex. Maybe the pain from having sex has made it less enjoyable? Psychological changes can also push the breaks on desire. Anxiety, depression, stress, and poor body image can occur in midlife and make sex seem less appealing. It's important to address all of these issues and not only look at falling estrogen and testosterone levels, so make check this list and mark off what you think might be affecting your desire for sex:

Physical

- Vaginal dryness
- Painful sex
- Fatigue
- Hot flashes
- Incontinence
- Chronic pain
- Side effects from medication

Psychological

- Anxiety/Depression
- Stress
- Poor body image
- Low self-esteem
- History of sexual trauma
- Substance abuse
- Side effects from medication (especially birth control pills and antidepressants)

Relationship

- Relationship difficulties
- Partner's sexual dysfunction

- Lack of available time together

If you are concerned that psychological or relationship issues are interfering with your ability to have sex, it's time to meet with someone who can help. A counselor or psychologist might be able to help you resolve some of these things that are turning you off. If side effects from medication are a concern, don't be afraid to be open with your health care provider about how it might be affecting your sex life. There might be an alternative. For the rest, keep reading and we will get into some natural treatments for some of the other physical issues resulting from menopause that are impeding on your sex life.

The Dry Vagina Monologues

Do you remember when the play, *The Vagina Monologues* came out? People were shocked that women were openly talking about their vaginas and sexuality. Well let's talk about dry vaginas in this section because a dry vagina is an unhappy vagina.

Just as they did as they transitioned through puberty, every woman will experience vulvar and vaginal changes as they transition through menopause too. When estrogen levels drop, the vulvar and vaginal tissues become thinner, drier, and less elastic. Because of this, it's common to suffer from burning, itching, irritation, and even spotting or bleeding. Sex can be painful. Although a change in hormones is a very common reason why your vagina might be uncomfortable, you should always show up to your annual check-up at your gynecologist's office. Other reasons why your vagina might be on vacation include:

- Bacterial or yeast Infections. They can become problematic as there may be a change in the vaginal flora, the community of helpful bacteria and other microorganisms living in your vagina.
- Allergic reactions to soap, laundry detergent, lotion, condoms, or feminine hygiene products

- Sexually transmitted infections such as herpes, genital warts, gonorrhea, or trichomoniasis
- Vulvar or vaginal cancer
- Radiation from cancer treatment
- Vulvodynia, chronic pain around the vaginal opening

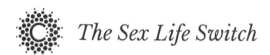

The Sex Life Switch

SWITCH #1 Lifestyle Changes

Ditch the douche. Vaginal douches alter the acidity of your vagina and when it isn't balanced, the vaginal flora (bacteria and yeast that live in your vagina) get out of whack, putting you at a higher risk for dryness, burning, itchiness, irritation, and infection.

Moisturize. Vaginal moisturizers are sold over-the-counter but there are also natural options such as vitamin E or olive oil, which you can rub directly onto the vulva and vagina several times a week to help with dryness. Do not use other oils as they may cause problems. Vaginal moisturizers are not applied directly before sex, vaginal lubricants are, so read below.

Lube up. Vaginal lubricants are also sold over-the-counter and are applied directly before sex or during sex. Not all lubes are created equal. I recommend you only use water-based lubricants and avoid these toxic chemicals as they may increase the risk of infection, reproductive problems, and/or cancer:

- Chlorhexidine gluconate
- Parabens (methlyparaben and/or propylparaben)
- Cyclomethicone, cyclopentasiloxane, and cyclotetrasiloxane, found in silicone-based
- Artificial flavors and fragrances

Lubricants containing petroleum jelly or mineral oil should also be avoided as they can increase your risk of infection. Oil-based lubricants are also not safe to use with latex condoms.

Avoid Irritants. Skip the bubble baths because soap doesn't belong in your vagina. You should only wash your vaginal area with warm water. Using soap strips away the healthy, protective vaginal flora as well as natural oils. Choose laundry detergent designed for sensitive skin so your underwear is free from irritating chemicals, avoid using moistened wipes, perfumes, fabric softeners, and scented toilet paper.

Pelvic floor exercises (Kegels). If you love your vagina, give her a squeeze. Kegels can increase blood flow to your vagina and strengthen vaginal wall muscles, which are involved in orgasm. Practice contracting your vaginal muscles for up to 10 seconds at a time with 10 second breaks, three times a day.

Use it or lose it. Regular sex can increase blood flow to your vagina and maintain healthy tissues. Your vagina can lose elasticity if you don't use it. Of course, don't use it if it's painful. You need to treat that problem first so you can enjoy sex.

Exercise. Increasing blood flow isn't only good for your brain and heart, it's good for your vagina too.

Avoid smoking and alcohol. Another good reason to stop smoking is because it reduces blood flow to your vagina. Alcohol slows down sexual response, making it harder to become lubricated and also orgasm. A glass of wine might put you in the mood but it's harder to enjoy sex once it's happening.

Let loose. Avoid tightfitting pantyhose and nylon underwear as these can restrict airflow and retain moisture, putting you at a higher risk for infections. Find something sexy in cotton.

Adjust your attitude. Start by being positive. Think about what turns you on about your partner and what you enjoy in bed. Don't think of sex as a chore but rather an enjoyment, a break from the hustle and bustle of daily life and a way of connecting with your inner self.

Communicate and Connect. Talking with your partner about what you do or don't like in bed can be stressful for most couples. The truth is that you should be connected enough to be able to have this conversation without worrying about what the other thinks. Don't judge when your partner tells you his or her desires or fears. Take time to listen and share yours as well. By doing this you will become more intimate with each other and your sexual relationship will become stronger.

Make your partner a priority. Take time for each other. Go on regular dates. Put your partner first by focusing on what makes him or her tingle. Offer a sensual massage, cook a nice dinner, and go for a long walk together. Make your partner feel like a top priority and you will mostly likely find it reciprocated.

Make sex a priority. Busy, stressful lives can put a damper on your sex life if you don't make time for it. The key word is "making" time. Plan a romantic overnight trip or staycation at home to relax and focus on each other. As unsexy as it sounds, putting sex on the schedule may be the key to an exhilarating sex life.

SWITCH #2 Supplements

DHEA. An over-the-counter DHEA supplement can boost testosterone levels which may improve libido. Taking a low dose of 10 mg per day of DHEA has been shown to increase sexual desire in postmenopausal women [61]. Start with 5 mg and see if it has an effect before increasing it to 10 mg. I never recommend taking DHEA without monitoring by a health care provider so levels don't become too high. Most men take 25 mg to 100 mg of DHEA and that is too much for most women, which can lead to unwanted effects including hair loss, body hair growth, greasy hair, greasy skin, and acne.

Maca. As mentioned in an earlier section, maca is a native South American plant that has been found to be especially helpful for improving sexual desire in postmenopausal women, possibly by raising estrogen levels [62]. Maca may also help with vaginal dryness. A common dose is 2,000 mg per day.

Vitamin E. Taking a vitamin E supplement of 50 to 400 IU per day by mouth for at least four weeks can increase blood supply to the vaginal wall to help with dryness. You can also apply vitamin E directly to your vagina to help with dryness. There are vitamin E suppositories sold over-the-counter for convenience.

Zinc. Oysters don't get their reputation as an aphrodisiac for no reason. They are very rich in zinc (6 medium oysters provide 32 mg, or 291% of the DV). It's better to get zinc from food than taking a supplement but if you do, don't take more than 50 mg per day as too much zinc can be harmful. It should also be taken in combination with copper, close to a 10:1 ratio (10 mg zinc with 1 mg copper).

CHAPTER 13
HAIR, SKIN, & NAILS

"I think that ultimately your age is determined by your attitude. It's not the number; it's not how many wrinkles you have on your face. It's the energy that you project."
—Christie Brinkley

Unwanted Hair Growth: The Bearded Lady

We all want thick, beautiful hair. Unfortunately, it ends up in places we don't want it to be as we transition to menopause. Hirsutism is a condition of unwanted male-pattern hair growth in women and can happen in midlife. This can affect the upper lip, chin, sideburns, inner thighs, chest, and the "happy trail" that runs from your belly button to your pubic area. There are more midlife women who come to my clinic for laser hair removal on their upper lip and chin than anywhere else on their bodies. These little rogue hairs are usually the result of the same hormone imbalance that causes acne to pop up: testosterone takes the reigns while estrogen rides in the back seat.

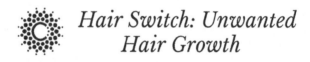

Hair Switch: Unwanted Hair Growth

SWITCH #1 Supplements

Diindolylmethane (DIM) is a phytonutrient derived from cruciferous vegetables such as broccoli, cauliflower, Brussels sprouts, cabbage, and kale. It blocks androgen receptors which makes it quite effective for both acne and hair growth in places you don't want it. I recommend 100 mg per day. Higher amounts could have unwanted effects (i.e. hot flashes) since it can decrease estrogen.

Saw palmetto is a palm that grows in the southeastern United States and may lower testosterone, which can help with unwanted male-pattern hair growth. A common dosage is 160 mg per day.

Spearmint tea (*Mentha spicata*). One study found that women with hirsutism who drank one cup of spearmint tea twice a day had lower levels of testosterone [63]. The researchers thought the tea might reduce symptoms of mild hirsutism. Another study found that spearmint tea lowered androgen levels in women who had PCOS [64].

Zinc decreases testosterone and increases progesterone, which may reduce male-pattern hair growth in women. It also inhibits the enzyme 5 alpha-reductase, which reduces the conversion of testosterone to dihydrotestosterone (DHT), a hormone that in high amounts is responsible for female-pattern hair loss. As mentioned in an earlier section, it's better to get zinc from food. However, research suggests taking 30 to 50 mg with a meal improves hirsutism after eight weeks [65]. Don't take zinc on an empty stomach, or it could make you feel sick.

SWITCH #2 Hair Removal

If laser hair removal isn't an option for you, there are plenty of other ways to get rid of these little stragglers. Waxing, plucking, electrolysis, bleaching, and shaving are common techniques. If you have heard that you shouldn't shave facial hair because it will grow back thicker, don't worry! It is only an old wives' tale. Hairs are thinner on the top and thicker on the bottom, so when you cut a hair with a razor blade at the bottom, it only looks thicker but I assure you that the hairs are actually not any thicker than before. Also, plucking gray hairs do not cause more gray hairs to grow. In fact, the more you pluck the less likely it will grow back because you damage the hair follicle each time. Same goes for waxing. So, if you want to avoid bald spots on your head, don't pick gray hairs out. But if you want to create bald spots on your chin, keep plucking and waxing them.

Tumbleweed blowing in the wind: Hair Loss

Almost 70% of women will experience thinning hair or bald spots as they transition through menopause. Female pattern hair loss, also called androgenic alopecia, occurs when the hair's growing phase slows down and it also takes longer for new hairs to begin growing. The hair follicles (little pockets in the skin that grow hairs) shrink and as a result the hairs become thinner and easily broken. This happens with age, an imbalance in hormones, or it can result from thyroid disease, chronic stress, genetics, poor health habits, and certain medications. If you have been evaluated by a health care provider and serious medical conditions have been ruled out, there are some natural treatments you can attempt at home to support healthy hair.

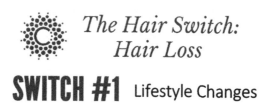

The Hair Switch:
Hair Loss

SWITCH #1 Lifestyle Changes

Hair Care. To prevent damage, you need to nurture the protective layer around your hair strands that keeps it shiny and flexible. When hair becomes dried out, this protective layer is destroyed and your hair looks dull and frizzy and it easily breaks, contributing to hair loss and split ends. Use organic hair dyes when coloring your hair and try to choose a natural color that is easy to maintain so you don't have to color your hair frequently. Let your hair air dry or use a low setting when using a hair dryer or curling iron. Use a wide-tooth comb to detangle before using a brush with more bristles, to prevent breakage. Shampoo your hair as less as possible and always use a moisturizing conditioner. If your skin and hair are dry (often due to low estrogen or thyroid), there's no need to shampoo your hair often since the scalp doesn't become oily.

Smoking cigarettes lowers estrogen in the body, which can contribute to dry hair that easily breaks.

Nutrition. Iron deficiency is the world's most common nutritional deficiency and a contributing factor for hair loss. Deficiencies of zinc, niacin, omega-3 and omega-6 fatty acids, selenium, vitamins A, D, E, folic acid, and biotin have all been linked to hair loss [66]. Eating a wide variety of foods and making sure your protein intake is adequate is important for healthy hair.

Stress reduction. Although not all hair loss is caused by stress, high stress levels can contribute to hair loss and thinning hair. Practicing stress reduction techniques such as exercise, breathing exercises, meditation, and gratitude journaling may not only help you feel better, but it will also help your hair grow better.

50 Shades of Gray...Hair

Gray hairs are inevitable and there's no magic porridge that can stop your golden locks from fading into 50 shades of gray. Our hair follicles make less melanin (pigment) as we age. Smoking, chronic stress, poor nutrition, chronic illness, and obesity have been found to speed up the process. However, genetics also play a role so if your parents were prematurely gray (20 to 30 years old), there's a strong possibility you followed the same footsteps.

SWITCH #2 Supplements

Because supplements for general hair, skin, and nail health are so interrelated, check out the end of this chapter for the master list.

Nails

Take a look at your fingernails. Are they smooth and perfectly rounded with a healthy pink glow? Or do you have to resort to applying fake nails or slathering on nail polish to cover up your unsightly fingernail problems? As you go through menopause, you may notice that your nails seem drier and more brittle than usual. Any new changes in your nails can be caused by lower estrogen levels, which can lead to dehydration. Like your skin, your nails need moisture.

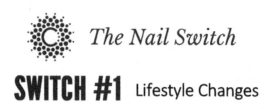

The Nail Switch

SWITCH #1 Lifestyle Changes

Nail Care. Wearing gloves when your hands are in water, such as when doing the dishes or washing the car, can protect your nails. If your nails are submerged in water for a long time, they absorb a lot of water, then contract as they dry out, damaging your nails. This is worsened if you are using strong soap. Keeping your nails moisturized will also help. There are nail moisturizers sold in the nail polish section that you can use. These are usually made of oil.

Smoking. You don't paint your nails yellow so why would you want to stain them with it? I often find that nothing gets through to a woman better than her own vanity. So... Let me tell you this: Smoking doesn't only have serious consequences to your health, it can ruin your skin, hair, and nails and make you look like a wretch. Just quit. The mirror on the wall will thank you.

Nutrition. If you want healthy fingernails, you have to nourish yourself from the inside-out. Dry, brittle nails are often caused by a deficiency in B-complex vitamins, especially biotin, which will produce ridges along the nail bed. A diet lacking in calcium and omega 3 also contributes to dry, brittle nails. Got hangnails? A lack of folic acid and vitamin C can lead to this.

Fight the Fungus. My go-to for treating toenail fungus is by rubbing tea tree oil on the nail. Although the evidence that supports the use of tea tree oil for treating nail fungus is limited, I have personally used it and it worked. It just takes time. Hold a tea tree oil-soaked cotton ball against the affected nail for several minutes. Do this daily for at least several weeks and make sure you keep your toenails as clean and dry as possible.

SWITCH #2 Supplements

Because supplements for general hair, skin, and nail health are so interrelated, check out the end of this chapter for the master list.

The Skinny on Midlife Skin

Your skin is your body's largest organ and a direct reflection of your internal health and your age. As you get older and you experience a drop in hormones, your skin becomes drier and less elastic. Within the first five years of menopause, you will lose about 30 percent of the collagen in your skin, making it look more wrinkled. Brown spots may start to appear on your skin, especially over areas that were the most exposed to the sun throughout the years. You may not be able to erase all of the damage, but there are things you can do that may make a significant improvement and slow down the signs of aging.

Acne: Return with a Vengeance

Many women are surprised when their skin retaliates against them in middle age. What was once in the past has unexpectedly returned. Acne in midlife is caused by a change in hormone balance. As estrogen drops, sometimes the testosterone train is still chugging, with a boxcar of pimples lugging behind it. One out of four women will suffer from midlife acne and it can take about five years for it to subside (when your ovaries make less testosterone). However, if you are struggling with it, I recommend seeing a dermatologist so you don't end up with scarring, since skin doesn't heal as well during older age.

Age Spots: Mark of the Menopausal Beast

Estrogen plays a role in the production of melanin, a dark pigment that is found in hair, skin, and eyes but is also responsible for tanning. Estrogen regulates its production and keeps it under control. As estrogen levels fall during menopause, melanin can take the reins and in areas of the skin that have been exposed to UV rays over the years, brown "age spots" start appearing on the face, hands, neck, arms and chest of many women.

If you are reading this book, you are probably from the Coppertone generation, when women doused themselves in baby oil while laying on plastic beach chairs between the 1970's and 1980's. Little was known about the harsh effects of the sun and promenading around in bronzed skin represented health and youth. Now, we know the reality of sun worshiping. Research shows that UV exposure is the reason behind 80% of your skin's aging. Not to mention, melanoma is the fastest growing cancer in the U.S. and worldwide.

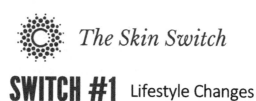

The Skin Switch

SWITCH #1 Lifestyle Changes

Sun Protection. I'm not opposed to a healthy amount of sunlight. Moderate sun exposure is good for your bones, immune system, and mood. However, this means about 10 minutes a day, not sizzling on the beach for hours until you become a fried egg. Apply up to SPF 30 to areas of the skin that have the most exposure to the sun (shoulders, face) if you are going to be in the sun for longer periods of time.

> **A note on sunless tanning:** I always questioned if sunless tanning is really a better alternative to sunbathing. I was never a fan of sunless tanning and I am still not. Replacing the sun by spraying chemicals all over your body doesn't sound like a great alternative. Because sunless tanning is a relatively new thing,

there is very little research about its effects, specifically with its main ingredient, dihydroxyacetone (DHA). It was thought that DHA was not significantly absorbed through the skin, but now it's believed that about 11% is absorbed deep into the dermis, a deep layer of the skin that contains blood capillaries, which may absorb DHA and spread it throughout the rest of the body. Other additives in sunless tanning products may contain hormone disrupting chemicals. In addition, some scientists have expressed concern that repeated exposure to spray tans may cause health problems due to inhalation of DHA, including the risk of asthma, COPD, and lung cancer.

Sleep. They didn't give Sleeping Beauty her name without reason. A good night's sleep can mean good skin health because when you're sleep-deprived, your body makes more of the stress hormone cortisol. Elevated levels of cortisol can lead to increased stress and inflammation in the body, hurting your skin's quality. In addition, while you're sleeping, the body's hydration rebalances. Skin is able to recover moisture, while excess water in general in the body is processed for removal. Not getting enough sleep results in poor water balance, leading to puffy bags under your eyes and under-eye circles, as well as dryness and more visible wrinkles. Lastly, during deep sleep, the rise in growth hormones allows damaged cells to become repaired. Without the deeper phases of sleep, this won't occur, allowing daily small breakdowns to accumulate instead of being reversed overnight. This results in more noticeable signs of aging. So, get your 8 hours in if you want to wake up looking like a princess.

Feed your face with fruits and veggies. Like, literally. A healthy diet rich in fresh fruits and vegetables means plenty of antioxidants to go to war against skin aging. The best way to be beautiful on the outside means working on it from the inside.

Smoking. The nicotine in cigarettes causes narrowing of the blood vessels, which impairs blood flow to your skin. With less blood flow, your skin doesn't get as much oxygen and important nutrients. To make matters worse, many of the more than 4,000 chemicals in tobacco smoke also damage collagen and elastin, which are fibers that give your skin its strength and elasticity. As a result, skin begins to sag and wrinkle.

Skin Care. Moisturize, moisturize, moisturize! You should be moisturizing your skin at least once per day, preferably twice per day. Make sure you have two moisturizers on hand: one for your face and one for your body. Even better, buy an eye cream as well because the skin pores around your eye area are smaller than those found on the rest of your body so if you rub body cream around your eyes, it won't absorb well.

Drink up. It is important to keep hydrated as the lack of estrogen in your body means that you cannot retain water as effectively as before. The more hydrated you are, the better your skin will look.

Maintain a healthy weight. Being overweight or obese can wreak havoc on your hormones, contributing to skin that is oily and acne-prone.

SWITCH #2 Face Lift in a Bottle

Okay, so I can't promise drastic results, but there are some over-the-counter creams and lotions that may provide modest benefits for more youthful skin. Just make sure you practice patience because better skin doesn't happen over the night. You will most likely need to use these for weeks or months before you notice an improvement. Look for topical skin care products that contain these ingredients:

Caffeine. Gives skin a firmer appearance by constricting blood vessels. It also has antioxidant properties that can slow down the process of photoaging (sun damage).

Coenzyme Q10. An antioxidant that reduces the appearance of wrinkles and fine lines by helping the skin produce more collagen and elastin.

Grape Seed Extract and Resveratrol. Delivers vitamin E, a nutrient that concentrates in the membranes of **skin** cells and helps hold on to moisture.

Hydroxy Acids. Smooth, tighten, firm and brighten the skin by weakening the 'cellular glue' that makes dead skin cells stick together, encouraging exfoliation and revealing healthy, younger skin cells.

Hyaluronic acid. A powerful moisturizer that reduces the appearance of fine lines and wrinkles and speeds up wound healing.

Kojic acid. Lightens visible sun damage, age spots, or scars.

Niacinamide (Vitamin B3). Increases the production of ceramides, which protect your skin barrier and seal in moisture. Also improves discoloration, repairs damage and neutralizes free radicals that can cause skin cancer and the breakdown of collagen and elastin.

Peptides. Signal the body to produce more collagen, reducing the appearance of wrinkles and fine lines.

Plant Stem Cells. Work by replacing, instead of repairing, damaged cells in the skin. Increases collagen production and reduces inflammation.

Retinol. Made from vitamin A, it boosts the amount of collagen your body makes and plumps out skin, reducing fine lines and wrinkles. It also improves skin tone and color and reduces mottled patches.

Tea extracts. Possess potent antioxidant and skin-soothing properties. Improves the appearance of sun-damaged skin and may protect you from skin cancer.

Vitamin C. One of the most potent antioxidants available, it brightens, firms, and protects your skin.

Vitamin E. A powerful antioxidant that reduces inflammation on your skin.

Vitamin K. Helps to reverse the appearance of aging in skin because of its role in blood circulation, making it perfect for under-eye creams.

Hair, Skin, and Nail Supplements

Biotin is a water-soluble vitamin that's also known as vitamin H or B7. It plays an important role in the health of your hair, skin, and nails. If you aren't getting enough biotin, you may experience hair loss. In most cases, the biotin you get from your diet is enough and deficiencies are rare. Foods rich in biotin include organ meats such as liver or kidney, egg yolks, and nuts. There isn't a lot of research that supports taking an oral biotin supplement unless you truly suffer from a deficiency, however a couple studies found that it may improve keratin, a protein that makes up hair, skin, and nails. The recommended dosage of biotin is up to 10 mg per day.

Healthy Fats. Essential fatty acids like omega-3s are the building blocks of healthy cell membranes. If you're not getting enough fatty acids in your diet, your skin may be dry and inflamed, your nails may look dry and brittle, and your hair may look dry and break easily. Fatty fish such as salmon and mackerel, flax seeds, chia seeds, and walnuts are excellent sources of omega-3. Taking a fish or krill oil supplement also packs a punch. Start with 1,000mg per day.

Did You Know?
The quality of fish oil/omega 3 greatly matters. It should be made from ocean fish from cold water (north Atlantic), not the fish hatchery! Most of the fish oil sold cheap or in bulk are poor quality and useless.

Iron. Iron is necessary for making red blood cells. When iron levels are low, the skin, hair, and nails don't get enough oxygen to stay healthy. Hair may become dry, lack shine, and even begin to fall out. The skin can look pale, dull, and may bruise easily and nails can appear dry and brittle. Iron rich foods include spinach, peas, and lean proteins. Iron is better absorbed when combined with vitamin C so load up on more oranges, strawberries, broccoli, and tomatoes. You can also take an iron supplement but don't take more than recommended because your body stores it and it can be a problem if levels become too high. I don't usually recommend that menopausal women take an iron supplement unless they have a poor diet because it's not often needed since they no longer have monthly bleeding which is when iron needs are higher, so it's best to check with your doctor first.

Probiotic. There is some evidence that taking probiotics might help to prevent or treat certain skin conditions such as acne, rosacea, and eczema, and may help to build collagen which improves texture and tone. To me, this is absolute no-brainer. Yes, I am going to bring up cave people again. Think about it – Our skin has been exposed to bacteria for millions of years. If you take away the beneficial bacteria, like we do in modern times, your skin suffers. Adult acne is on the rise, along with other skin conditions. Yes, I am sure stress and exposure to toxins in our environment also play a role, but I think the lack of exposure to bacteria also has its part. Some probiotic strains found to be effective in studies of acne include Lactobacillus, L. acidophilus, and B. bifudum. Good sources of probiotics include yogurt, kefir, kombucha, kimchi, sauerkraut, and miso.

Did You Know?
Flavored yogurts are often packed with sugar. It is better to buy plain Greek yogurt (which has more protein than regular yogurt) and top it off with fresh fruit or preserves with no added sugar.

Resveratrol. This is an antioxidant powerhouse. Resveratrol is in the spotlight in the research world for everything from cancer to brain disease to skin disorders. It can be found in cosmetic products but if you want wide benefits of this super-antioxidant, a supplement may be what you need. Resveratrol is the key ingredient that makes red wine heart healthy. To save yourself from drinking copious amounts of calories and alcohol, you can also take a supplement. Use with caution if you have a blood clotting disorder or are on blood thinners.

Vitamin C. A deficiency in vitamin C can result in brittle nails, as well as slowed nail growth. Vitamin C is essential for collagen production, which helps provide strength and integrity to your nails. *Some research suggests* that *vitamin C* may help prevent and treat ultraviolet (UV)-induced photodamage. Normal *skin* contains high concentrations of *vitamin C*, which supports important and well-known functions, stimulating collagen synthesis. Citrus fruits, broccoli, and spinach are great food sources of vitamin C. If you take a supplement, make sure it is buffered with minerals so it doesn't upset your stomach and it is better absorbed.

Vitamin D helps skin cells grow and repair, which prevents skin aging. Vitamin D also stimulates hair follicles to grow. Vitamin D deficiency may be linked to alopecia areata, an autoimmune condition that causes patchy hair loss. A deficiency may also cause peeling nails. Many women are deficient in vitamin D, especially after menopause because estrogen increases the activity of an enzyme responsible for activating vitamin D. There are not many foods very rich in vitamin D. Salmon and swordfish are food sources but most people don't get enough vitamin D through diet. Healthy sun exposure is your best bet. You can also take a supplement.

Vitamin E. Vitamin E helps block free radicals from damaging your skin, helping prevent wrinkles and protecting your collagen and elastin from breaking down — a very important factor that can cause premature aging. Foods rich in vitamin E include olive oil, almonds, lean meats and leafy greens. Personally, I take a vitamin E (400IU) supplement every day. Use with caution if you are on blood thinners.
Zinc. While most of us get a sufficient amount of zinc from our diet, zinc deficiency can cause hair loss. Zinc can improve hair growth in people who are deficient in it. Zinc has also shown to have anti-inflammatory properties and can help reduce the amount of acne-causing bacteria in the skin and treat inflamed acne. It's better to get zinc from food (such as oysters) than taking a supplement but if you

do, don't take more than 50 mg per day as too much zinc can be harmful. It should also be taken in combination with copper, close to a 10:1 ratio (10 mg zinc with 1 mg copper).

Collagen: The Scoop on Bone Soup. A new wave of edible collagen products is flooding the market, such as powders, which you can add to coffee or smoothies and pills that you can take along with your morning multivitamin. However, collagen supplements are controversial and according to some Harvard University researchers [67], dietary collagen doesn't get transported directly to your skin because when you consume collagen, it gets broken down into amino acids during digestion. Your body then uses the amino acids to make new protein, which could go toward replenishing collagen, but they're actually more likely to go toward major muscles we need to function (e.g., your heart, diaphragm and brain) than to the crow's feet around your eyes. Because not enough is known, I cannot say yes or no for buying them but if you do, look for companies that get their bones and tissues from cage-free, free-range, and antibiotic-free sources. Look for a trusted brand with a third-party label like NSF or USP.

Epilogue

I never planned on writing a book. It sort of just came together.

As a student, I wrote health and wellness articles in my blog just out of pure satisfaction, like a nerdy hobby.

I was also dealing with my own hormonal problems and mainstream medicine just didn't offer a natural approach to the root cause of my problem. I had to find the solutions myself so I poured a ton of time and energy into it, and eventually found the golden ticket to heal myself.

When I became a practitioner, I started writing weekly emails to my patients about weight loss and hormones. Over time, I accumulated all of this stuff, all of this content, and I felt like I could do something more. A book, I thought, was a great way to help women. I could hand one out to every midlife woman who walks into my clinic, as well as others on the other side of the world. So I dove through my piles of content, spent about a year sifting through it, and digging into new research findings to create this book.

It wasn't easy. Almost as hard as writing my doctoral dissertation or having children. Although to be fair, I have always loved having kids, as if I was born to raise children. Like all mothers, I nurture them with love, but also know how to step back and watch them grow. I often say that kids are like orchids. They often bloom even if you stop watering them.

With that being said, as a conclusion for this book, I want to remind you that we, as women and as mothers, also need nurturing. Don't forget to water yourself. I gave you the seeds, which included a basic understanding of your hormones, what happens when they go awry, and steps to take to bring yourself back into balance. It's up to you to water yourself, to apply these techniques so that you can feel strong, vibrant, confident, and fabulous. I wish you a lot of bright and sunny days and a season of change. The best of days is yet to come.

Now is the time for you to tell me your story. I want you to share your unique journey with me. The best way to do that is to visit DoctorCarissa.com and send me a message. I'm looking forward to hearing from you.

PART FOUR

Recipes

A word from Chef Gui Alinat

I'm honored and proud to be contributing these awesome recipes to my wife's book, The Menopause Switch.

Cooking food to help your menopausal symptoms doesn't have to be bland and boring. It can be delicious. My goal was to create great tasting recipes that you will enjoy, in addition to reaping the full health benefits of the super nutrients Dr. Carissa put together for you.

The recipes we created revolve around a simple concept: Jam-pack them with lots of fruits and vegetables with a limited amount of meat or seafood. Avoid grains including corn, dairy, artificial sweeteners, soybeans, and peanuts, because they are inflammatory.

You'll find 7 breakfast, 7 lunch, 7 snack, and 7 dinner recipes. They are meant to be simple and quick. There is no need for you to spend more time in the kitchen than you actually want to.

So enjoy!

Raspberry-Grapefruit Smoothie
Active time: 5 minutes
Yield: 1 serving

Ingredients
Juice of 1 pink grapefruit
1 banana peeled and sliced
1/2 cup raspberries
1/2 cup blackberries or
blueberries

Preparation
Place all ingredients in a blender
and process until smooth.

Chia Berry Parfait
Active time: 10 minutes
Yield: 2 servings

Ingredients
1/4 cup chia seeds
1 cup coconut milk
1 tablespoon organic pure
maple syrup
1 teaspoon vanilla extract
1 cup organic granola
2 cups mixed berries

Preparation
In a mixing bowl, mix the chia seeds
with the milk, maple syrup and
vanilla extract. Divide into 2 serving
bowls. Cover, refrigerate, and let it
set overnight for the seeds to gel.
The next day, make the parfait: add
the granola and the berries on top of
the gelled chia seeds. Serve and
enjoy.

Moistest Chocolate & Zucchini Bread
Active time: 10 minutes
Cooking time: 50 minutes
Yield: 1 loaf

Ingredients
1 cup grated zucchini (about 1 small zucchini)
3/4 cup all-natural creamy almond butter
1/4 cup pure maple syrup
2 large eggs, slightly beaten
1/2 teaspoon vanilla extract
2 tablespoons coconut flour
1 teaspoon baking soda
1/2 teaspoon cinnamon
1/2 cup dark 80% cocoa chocolate, broken into small pieces

Preparation
Preheat oven to 350°F (180 C). Line an 8x4 inch loaf pan with parchment paper and brush a little extra-virgin olive oil.

In a large bowl, mix zucchini, almond butter, maple syrup, eggs and vanilla with whisk until well combined and creamy. Stir in coconut flour, baking soda and cinnamon. Mix until just combined. Next, fold in the chocolate.

Pour batter into loaf pan. Bake for 40-50 minutes or until a knife inserted in the bread comes out clean.

Chocolate Waffles

Active time: 30 minutes
Cooking time: 8 minutes
Yield: 2 waffles

Ingredients

3 eggs
1/4 cup coconut milk
1/4 cup coconut flour
1/4 cup unsweetened cacao powder
1/4 cup coconut sugar
¼ teaspoon baking soda
¼ teaspoon salt
1 tablespoon coconut oil

Preparation

Preheat a waffle maker. In a blender, add eggs, milk, coconut flour, cacao, coconut sugar, baking soda and salt. Process and pulse until you obtain a smooth batter. Ladle some of the batter into each waffle square. At this time, you also have the opportunity to add any additional ingredients such as dark chocolate chips. Scatter these over the top of the mixture. Close the lid and cook for approximately 4 minutes or until nice and crispy.

Omelet Muffins

Active time: 15 minutes
Cooking time: 20 minutes
Yield: 8 muffins

Ingredients

8 eggs
8 ounces cooked ham, crumbled
1 cup diced red bell pepper
1 cup diced onion
Salt and pepper to taste
2 tablespoons coconut milk

Preparation

Preheat oven to 350°F (180°C). Grease 8 muffin cups. Beat eggs together in a large bowl, and add ham, bell pepper, onion, salt and pepper and coconut milk into the beaten eggs. Pour egg mixture evenly into prepared muffin cups. Bake in the preheated oven until muffins are set in the middle, 18 to 20 minutes.

Coconut Pancakes

Active time: 5 minutes
Cooking time: 10 minutes
Yield: Makes 6

Ingredients

3 tablespoons coconut oil

1 tablespoon raw honey

3 large eggs

1/4 cup coconut milk

1/2 teaspoon vanilla extract

1/4 cup coconut flour, sifted

1/4 teaspoon cream of tartar

1/8 teaspoon baking soda

Salt to taste

Preparation

In a blender, process 2 tablespoons of coconut oil, honey, eggs, coconut milk and vanilla. Pulse to mix. Add coconut flour, cream of tartar, baking soda, salt, and blend until smooth. Do not overmix. In a non-stick skillet under medium-high heat, add a bit of coconut oil, and pour a small amount of batter to make a pancake. Cook it for about 2 minutes. Flip once the bottom is light brown and finish cooking. Repeat to finish the batter. Serve immediately with a drizzle of maple syrup.

Baked Eggs and Spinach

Active time: 15 minutes
Cooking time: 15 minutes
Yield: 4 servings

Ingredients

3 tablespoons extra-virgin olive oil
1 pound baby spinach
1 /2 onion, roughly chopped
1 clove garlic, minced
1 tablespoon coconut flour
1 /2 cup almond milk
3 ounces Neufchâtel cheese
Pinch of freshly grated nutmeg
4 eggs
Salt and pepper to taste

Preparation

Preheat the oven to 350°F (180°C). Heat 1 tablespoon of olive oil in a seasoned skillet over medium heat. Quickly wilt the spinach. Season with salt and pepper and place the spinach in a colander over a bowl to drain.

Add 2 tablespoons of oil to the pan. When hot, add the onion and garlic and cook over medium heat until the onion is translucent and tender, about 5 minutes. Add the flour and cook, stirring, for 1 minute. Gradually whisk in the milk and, while whisking constantly, bring to a boil, about 3 minutes. Add the Neufchâtel cheese, nutmeg, and salt and pepper. Once the sauce has thickened, remove it from the heat and continue to whisk for 1 minute more. When the spinach has cooled, squeeze out any excess liquid, coarsely chop, and add to the warm sauce. Stir well to combine. Spread the spinach mixture in an even layer in the bottom of a baking dish. Using a spoon, make 4 wells in the spinach for the eggs. Pour 1 egg into each well. Bake until the spinach is warmed through and the eggs are set and cooked to the desired degree of doneness, about 15 minutes. Serve warm.

Kale Chips
Active time: 10 minutes
Cooking time: 15 minutes
Yield: 6 servings

Ingredients

1 bunch kale
1 tablespoon extra-virgin olive oil
Salt and pepper to taste

Preparation

Preheat an oven to 350°F (180°C). Line a sheet pan with parchment paper. Remove the stems from the kale leaves and tear into bite size pieces. Wash and thoroughly dry kale with a salad spinner. Drizzle kale with olive oil and sprinkle with salt and pepper. Bake until the edges brown but are not burnt, about 15 minutes.

Carrot Sweet Potato Smoothie
Active time: 5 minutes
Yield: 1 serving

Ingredients

1/2 cup chopped carrots
1/2 cup chopped sweet potato
1/2 cup banana, sliced and frozen
1-cup almond milk
1/4 cup frozen, diced pineapple
2 tablespoons pistachio
1/4 teaspoon cinnamon
Pinch nutmeg

Preparation

Place all ingredients into a high-power blender and blend until smooth.

Hard Boiled Eggs
Active time: 5 minutes
Cooking time: 7 ½ minutes
Yield 4 servings

Ingredients
4 eggs
1-tablespoon vinegar

Preparation
Bring water and vinegar to a full rolling boil, in a saucepan over medium-high heat.
Add eggs carefully with a slotted spoon. Time 7 ½ minutes.
Remove eggs from the water with a slotted spoon, and put in a bowl. Let the eggs cool at room temperature, then refrigerate

Raspberry Smoothie
Active time: 3 minutes
Yield: 2 servings

Ingredients
2 cups raspberries
1 banana
1-cup Greek yogurt
1/4 cup orange juice
2 teaspoon of vanilla extract

Preparation
In a blender, pulse all ingredients together until smooth.
Serve at once.

Crunchy Garbanzo
Active time: 3 minutes
Cooking time: 20 minutes
Yield: 2 servings

Ingredients
1 small can garbanzo beans
2 teaspoons extra-virgin olive oil
1-teaspoon cumin
1-teaspoon paprika
1/2 teaspoon salt

Preparation
Drain garbanzo beans and dry them. Place in an ovenproof dish and mix with all other ingredients.
Bake 20 minutes at 425°F. Serve at once.

Celery Root Sticks
Active time: 5 minutes
Yield: 2 servings

Ingredients
1 celery root
1-tablespoon lime juice
1-tbsp fresh cilantro, chopped
1-teaspoon chili powder
Salt to taste

Preparation
Peel the celery and cut it into sticks.
Toss with lime juice and sprinkle with chopped cilantro, salt, and chili powder. Serve.

Lupini Bean Salad
Active time: 10 minutes
Cooking time: 10 minutes
Yield: 6 servings

Ingredients
1-tablespoon coconut oil
1 small red onion, chopped
1-tablespoon chili powder
1-teaspoon ground cumin
2 15-oz cans lupini, rinsed
1/2 cup salsa
1/2 tsp sea salt
1-tablespoon lime juice
2 tablespoons fresh cilantro
Optional: cooked chicken

Preparation
Heat oil in a large saucepan over medium heat. Add the red onion and cook until it begins to soften.
Add chili powder and cumin and cook for 1 minute. Keep stirring. Add the beans, salsa, and salt and bring to a boil. Reduce the heat and simmer for about 5 minutes.
Remove from heat and add the lime juice. Chill for 30 minutes Serve with cilantro garnish. Add strips of cooked chicken to increase the protein if desired.

Cucumber and Avocado Salad

Active time: 15 minutes

Yield: 4 servings

Ingredients

2 medium cucumbers, diced (skin on)

2 avocados, peeled, pitted, and diced

4 tablespoons chopped fresh cilantro

1 clove garlic, minced

2 tablespoons minced scallions

Salt and pepper to taste

1/4 large lemon

1 lime

Preparation

In a large mixing bowl, delicately combine cucumbers, avocados, and cilantro. Stir in garlic, scallions, salt, and pepper. Squeeze lemon and lime over the top, and toss. Cover, and refrigerate for 20 minutes. Plate and serve.

Super Quick Tuscan Tomato Salad

Active time: 10 minutes

Yield: 6 servings

Ingredients

2 pounds ripe tomatoes

Salt and pepper to taste

1 1/2 cups cooked cannellini beans (omit for Paleo)

(15 ounce can, drained and rinsed)

1/2 cup finely diced celery

1 small garlic clove, minced

1/2 cup crumbled feta (omit for Paleo)

2 tablespoons chopped fresh mint

2 tablespoons sherry vinegar

1/4 cup extra virgin olive oil

3 cups baby arugula

Preparation

Cut tomatoes into thick slices. Lay on a large platter. Sprinkle with salt and pepper. Top with beans (if using), celery, garlic, feta (if using), mint, and arugula. Drizzle with vinegar and olive oil. Serve.

Vegan Stir Fry

Active time: 15 minutes
Cooking time: 20 minutes
Yield 1 serving

Ingredients

1/2 onion, chopped
1 carrot, sliced thinly
1/2 bell pepper, sliced
1/2 red pepper, sliced
1 cup potatoes, diced
small
1/2 cup black beans from
a can, drained (omit for
Paleo)
1 jalapeno, sliced
Bragg Liquid Aminos,
optional broccoli
2 cups Spinach
12 Asparagus, cut into
sticks

Preparation

Add onion, potatoes and carrots to a large skillet and cook for a few minutes, covered.

Add bell pepper and red pepper and stir. Cook for a few minutes more. If veggies are sticking, put a little water in the pan.

Add beans, and jalapeno. Cook for a few more minutes.

Once the potatoes are warmed, add aminos and stir again.

Add spinach and asparagus and put lid on skillet, do not stir. Cook for about 5 more minutes.

Unrolled Cabbage Rolls

Active time: 20 minutes
Cooking time: 25 minutes
Yield: 6 servings

Ingredients

2 pounds ground beef
1 large onion, chopped
1 small head cabbage, chopped
1 (28 ounce) cans diced tomatoes
1/2 cup water
2 cloves garlic, minced
Salt and pepper to taste

Preparation

Heat a Dutch oven over medium-high heat. Cook and stir beef and onion in the hot Dutch oven until browned and crumbly, 5 to 7 minutes. Drain and discard grease. Add cabbage, tomatoes, water, garlic, salt, and pepper and bring to a boil. Cover Dutch oven, reduce heat, and simmer until cabbage is tender, about 25 minutes.

Skillet Cauliflower Steaks

Active time: 15 minutes
Cooking time: 20 minutes
Serves: 4

Ingredients

1 head cauliflower
Salt and pepper to taste
1-tablespoon curry powder
2 leaves sage, finely chopped
1-tablespoon olive oil
1 lemon Juice

Preparation

Slice the cauliflower through the center, keeping as much intact as possible. Season the "steaks" with salt, pepper, curry, and sage. Sprinkle with olive oil and lemon juice.
Heat a cast iron skillet over medium high heat. Add olive oil and place cauliflower carefully in the pan. Sear the cauliflower for about 10 minutes per side, until deeply golden.

Vegetarian Chili

Active time: 20 minutes
Cooking time: 30 minutes
Yield: 4 servings

Ingredients

1 lime
1 red onion, thinly sliced
Extra-virgin olive oil
1 large onion, chopped
4 garlic cloves, minced
2 teaspoons chili powder
2 teaspoons dried oregano
2 (15 ounce) cans beans, drained
1 (15 ounce) can diced tomatoes
Salt and pepper, to taste
Fresh cilantro, for garnish
Sour cream, for garnish

Preparation

Make the pickled onions: In a bowl, squeeze the lime juice, add the onion, and a large pinch of salt. Let rest for 20 minutes while you make the chili. Heat a Dutch oven over medium-high heat, then add the oil. Add the onion and sauté until softened. Add the garlic, chili powder and oregano and sauté until fragrant. Add the beans and tomatoes, salt and pepper, and simmer until the tomatoes break down, about 20 minutes. Serve with the pickled onion or any of the garnishes you enjoy. Add crushed tomatoes, salt, pepper and stir. Bring to a simmer, reduce heat to low, and simmer until flavors are blended, 10 minutes.

Chicken Carrot Casserole

Active time: 20 minutes
Cooking time: 20 minutes
Yield: 3 servings

Ingredients

2 tablespoons coconut oil
2 large carrots, peeled and
cut into 1-inch pieces
1 celery stalk, chopped
Sea salt
Freshly ground black pepper
3 cloves garlic, minced
1 1/2 pounds chicken breasts
or firm tofu (for vegetarians)
3 sprigs thyme
1 bay leaf
3/4 pounds baby potatoes,
skin on, quartered
3 cups vegetable broth
2 tablespoons parsley,
chopped

Preparation

Melt coconut oil in a large pot
over medium heat.
Add carrots, celery, and season
with salt and pepper.
Cook until the vegetables are
tender. About five minutes.
Add garlic and cook for 30
seconds. Add chicken (or tofu),
thyme, bay leaf, potatoes and
broth. Season with salt and
pepper.
Simmer and cook for 15 minutes
or until potatoes are tender and
chicken is not pink.
Shred the chicken with a fork (if
using) and return to the bowl.
Garnish with parsley.

Turmeric and Ginger Chicken

Active time: 30 minutes
Cooking time: 20 minutes
Yield: 4 servings

Ingredients

1-teaspoon turmeric
1-teaspoon crushed garlic
1/2 teaspoon salt
1-teaspoon fresh ginger root, grated
1 onion, peeled and diced
1-teaspoon mild chopped chili
½-cup fresh lime Juice
½-cup coconut oil
½ cup of organic chicken stock
4 chicken legs
4 whole zucchinis, cut into large chunks

Preparation

Prepare all marinade ingredients (First 7 ingredients). Place in a food blender and blend to a paste.
Rub equal amounts of the paste into each thigh.
Place thighs in a glass container. Add any remaining paste, cover, and store in the fridge for up to 24 hours.
Preheat oven to 375 degrees F. Add some coconut oil to a sauté pan and warm,
Place the thighs and zucchini in the pan and very lightly seal on both side, immediately transfer to an oven baking tray.
Warm the chicken stock and pour around the chicken and zucchini. Cover with parchment paper or a pan lid and bake for 20 mins.

Italian Sausage and Vegetable Soup
Active time: 10 minutes
Cooking time: 40 minutes
Yield: 6 servings

Ingredients
1-pound turkey sausage
1 clove garlic, minced
1-tablespoon extra-virgin olive oil
2 (14 ounce) cans chicken broth
1 (14.5 ounce) can Italian diced tomatoes
1 cup sliced carrots
1 (14.5 ounce) can great Northern beans, undrained
2 small zucchini, diced
2 cups spinach - packed, rinsed and torn
Salt and pepper to taste

Preparation
In a cast iron Dutch oven or large soup pot, brown sausage with garlic in the extra-virgin olive oil over medium high heat.
Stir in broth, tomatoes and carrots, and season with salt and pepper. Reduce heat, cover, and simmer 15 minutes. Stir in beans with liquid and zucchini.
Cover and simmer another 15 minutes, or until zucchini is tender. Remove from heat, and add spinach.
Stir. Soup is ready to serve after 5 minutes.

Roasted Chicken Thighs with Peaches, Basil and Ginger
Active time: 10 minutes
Cooking time: 20 minutes
Yield: 2 servings

Ingredients
3 peaches
1-pound boneless, skinless chicken thighs
1-tablespoon coconut oil
2 tablespoons dry sherry
2 tablespoons chopped fresh basil
2 garlic cloves, minced
1 inch long piece fresh ginger root, grated
Salt and pepper to taste

Preparation
Preheat oven to 400°F (200 C). Halve peaches, remove pits and slice fruit ½ inch thick.
In an ovenproof dish, toss all ingredients except basil. Roast for 20 minutes, or until chicken is cooked through and peaches are softened. Garnish with basil and serve.

Mango Salsa Grilled Salmon
Active time: 10 minutes
Cooking time: 8 minutes
Yield: 4 servings

Ingredients
4 (8-ounce) salmon fillets
2 mangoes, peeled and diced
2 tablespoons chopped red onion
2 tablespoons chopped fresh basil
2 teaspoons extra-virgin olive oil
1-teaspoon chili oil
Salt and pepper to taste

Preparation
Combine mango, onions, basil, and the oils. Cover and chill 1 hour.
On a hot grill, place fish and grill 4 minutes on each side or until fish flakes easily when tested with a fork. Serve with mango salsa.

Stuffed Peppers with Turkey and Vegetables
Active time: 20 minutes
Cooking time: 30 minutes
Yield: 4 servings

Ingredients
4 green peppers, tops removed, seeded
1-pound ground turkey
2 tablespoons extra-virgin olive oil
1/2 onion, diced
1 cup sliced mushrooms
1 zucchini, diced
1 red pepper, chopped
1 yellow pepper, chopped
1-cup fresh spinach
1 (14.5 ounce) can diced tomatoes, drained
1-tablespoon tomato paste

1-tablespoon dry oregano
Salt and pepper to taste

Preparation
Preheat oven to 350°F (175C). In a skillet over medium-high heat, cook the turkey in 1 tablespoon of oil until evenly brown. Set aside. Heat the remaining oil in the skillet, and cook onion, mushrooms, zucchini, red bell pepper, yellow bell pepper, and spinach until tender. Return turkey to the skillet. Mix in the tomatoes and tomato paste, and season with oregano, salt, and pepper. Stuff the green peppers with the skillet mixture. Place in an ovenproof dish, cover with foil, and bake for 30 minutes.

Place green peppers in a baking dish. Bake 30 minutes in the preheated oven.

Serve.

Butternut Squash Lasagna
Active time: 15 minutes
Cooking time: 45 minutes
Yield: 8 servings

Ingredients
1 lb. hot Italian
sausage, casing
removed
1 onion
3 cloves garlic,
minced
1 (15 ounce can)
tomato sauce
1/2 cup roasted red
peppers
1/4 cup coconut oil
Fresh basil to taste
1 small butternut
squash
Mozzarella cheese

Preparation
Preheat oven to 400°F (200 C). In a skillet
over medium-high heat, add the sausage,
onions, and garlic, and brown.
Meanwhile, peel the butternut squash.
Split the two halves in half, lengthwise,
and remove the seeds. Cut the squash
into planks, to imitate lasagna pasta
sheets.
Make the sauce by blending tomato
sauce, red peppers, coconut oil and basil
in a food processor or blender.
In an ovenproof baking dish, pour enough
sauce to lightly cover the bottom of the
dish. Next add the squash, trying not to
overlap the pieces, then spoon on the
sausage mixture, followed by the sauce.
Repeat until all your ingredients are used
up, trying to reserve enough sauce to
cover the top of the lasagna. If using, top
with cheese. Bake for 45 minutes, until
bubbly and with a crispy, browned top.
Let it rest before serving.

Appendix A

Body Mass Index (BMI) Chart for Adults

Obese (>30) Overweight (25–30) Normal (18.5–25) Underweight (<18.5)

HEIGHT in feet/inches and centimeters

WEIGHT		4'8"	4'9"	4'10"	4'11"	5'0"	5'1"	5'2"	5'3"	5'4"	5'5"	5'6"	5'7"	5'8"	5'9"	5'10"	5'11"	6'0"	6'1"	6'2"	6'3"	6'4"	6'5"
lbs	(kg)	142cm		147	150	152	155	157	160	163	165	168	170	173	175	178	180	183	185	188	191	193	196
260	(117.9)	58	56	54	53	51	49	48	46	45	43	42	41	40	38	37	36	35	34	33	32	32	31
255	(115.7)	57	55	53	51	50	48	47	45	44	42	41	40	39	38	37	36	35	34	33	32	31	30
250	(113.4)	56	54	52	50	49	47	46	44	43	42	40	39	38	37	36	35	34	33	32	31	30	30
245	(111.1)	55	53	51	49	48	46	45	43	42	41	40	38	37	36	35	34	33	32	31	31	30	29
240	(108.9)	54	52	50	48	47	45	44	43	41	40	39	38	36	35	34	33	33	32	31	30	29	28
235	(106.6)	53	51	49	47	46	44	43	42	40	39	38	37	36	35	34	33	32	31	30	29	29	28
230	(104.3)	52	50	48	46	45	43	42	41	39	38	37	36	35	34	33	32	31	30	30	29	28	27
225	(102.1)	50	49	47	45	44	43	41	40	39	37	36	35	34	33	32	31	31	30	29	28	27	27
220	(99.8)	49	48	46	44	43	42	40	39	38	37	36	34	33	32	32	31	30	29	28	27	27	26
215	(97.5)	48	47	45	43	42	41	39	38	37	36	35	34	33	32	31	30	29	28	28	27	26	25
210	(95.3)	47	45	44	42	41	40	38	37	36	35	34	33	32	31	30	29	28	28	27	26	26	25
205	(93.0)	46	44	43	41	40	39	37	36	35	34	33	32	31	30	29	29	28	27	26	26	25	24
200	(90.7)	45	43	42	40	39	38	37	35	34	33	32	31	30	30	29	28	27	26	26	25	24	24
195	(88.5)	44	42	41	39	38	37	36	35	33	32	31	31	30	29	28	27	26	26	25	24	24	23
190	(86.2)	43	41	40	38	37	36	35	34	33	32	31	30	29	28	27	26	26	25	24	24	23	23
185	(83.9)	41	40	39	37	36	35	34	33	32	31	30	29	28	27	27	26	25	24	24	23	23	22
180	(81.6)	40	39	38	36	35	34	33	32	31	30	29	28	27	27	26	25	24	24	23	22	22	21
175	(79.4)	39	38	37	35	34	33	32	31	30	29	28	27	26	26	25	24	24	23	22	22	21	21
170	(77.1)	38	37	36	34	33	32	31	30	29	28	27	27	26	25	24	24	23	22	22	21	21	20
165	(74.8)	37	36	34	33	32	31	30	29	28	27	27	26	25	24	24	23	22	22	21	21	20	20
160	(72.6)	36	35	33	32	31	30	29	28	27	27	26	25	24	24	23	22	22	21	21	20	19	19
155	(70.3)	35	34	32	31	30	29	28	27	27	26	25	24	24	23	22	22	21	20	20	19	19	18
150	(68.0)	34	32	31	30	29	28	27	27	26	25	24	23	23	22	22	21	20	20	19	19	18	18
145	(65.8)	33	31	30	29	28	27	26	25	24	23	23	22	21	21	20	20	19	19	18	18	17	
140	(63.5)	31	30	29	28	27	26	26	25	24	23	23	22	21	21	20	20	19	18	18	17	17	17
135	(61.2)	30	29	28	27	26	25	25	24	23	22	22	21	21	20	19	19	18	18	17	17	16	16
130	(59.0)	29	28	27	26	25	25	24	23	22	22	21	20	20	19	19	18	18	17	17	16	16	15
125	(56.7)	28	27	26	25	24	24	23	22	21	21	20	20	19	18	18	17	17	16	16	16	15	15
120	(54.4)	27	26	25	25	23	23	22	21	21	20	19	19	18	18	17	17	16	16	15	15	15	14
115	(52.2)	26	25	24	23	22	22	21	20	20	19	19	18	17	17	16	16	16	15	15	14	14	14
110	(49.9)	25	24	23	22	21	21	20	19	19	18	18	17	17	16	16	15	15	15	14	14	13	13
105	(47.6)	24	23	22	21	20	19	19	18	17	17	16	16	16	15	15	14	14	13	13	13	12	
100	(45.4)	22	22	21	20	20	19	18	18	17	17	16	16	15	15	14	14	14	13	13	12	12	12
95	(43.1)	21	21	20	19	19	18	17	17	16	16	15	15	14	14	14	13	13	13	12	12	12	11
90	(40.8)	20	19	19	18	18	17	16	16	15	15	14	14	13	13	13	12	12	12	11	11	11	
85	(38.6)	19	18	18	17	17	16	16	15	15	14	14	13	13	13	12	12	12	11	11	11	10	10
80	(36.3)	18	17	17	16	16	15	15	14	14	13	13	13	12	12	11	11	11	11	10	10	10	9

NOTE: BMI values rounded to the nearest whole number. BMI categories based on CDC (Centers for Disease Control and Prevention) criteria.
BMI = weight(kg) / (height(m) x height(m)) = 703 x weight(lbs) / (height(in) x height(in))

DR. CARISSA

161

Appendix B

9 Health Screenings All Women Should Have

Health Concern	Recommendation
Blood Pressure	The American Heart Association (AHA) recommends that if your blood pressure is below 120/80, you should have it checked at least once every two years, beginning at age 20. For adults at a higher risk for high blood pressure (age 40 or older, African-American, obese), the United States Preventive Services Task Force (USPSTF) recommends it yearly.
Breast Cancer	The American Cancer Society recommends women have mammograms starting at 45, and can then switch to a biannual mammogram at age 55.
Cervical Cancer	A PAP test should be done every 3 years beginning at age 21 until age 65, according to the USPSTF.
Cholesterol	The AHA recommends that all adults 20 or older have their cholesterol checked every four to six years. After age 40, your health care provider will also want to use an equation to calculate your 10-year risk of experiencing cardiovascular disease or stroke.
Colon Cancer and polyps	A colonoscopy is recommended for women age 50 and older every 10 years.

Dental Health	All adult women should have twice-yearly dental checkups and cleanings.
Diabetes	A blood sugar screening is recommended for women aged 40 to 70 years who are overweight or obese.
Osteoporosis	A bone density test is recommended for women age 65 and older.
Skin Cancer	Women should examine their skin every month at home, according to the American Cancer Society.

These recommendations are based on healthy women. Your health care provider will recommend how often you should have these screenings.

Works Cited

1. American Thyroid Association. [Online] [Cited: November 8, 2019.] https://www.thyroid.org/media-main/press-room/.

2. Why is depression more prevalent in women? Albert, P.R. 4, 2015, Journal of Psychiatry and Neuroscience, Vol. 40, pp. 219-221.

3. The Croonian Lectures: On the chemical correlations of the functions of the body. Starling, E.H. s.l. : Lancet, 1905, Vol. 166, pp. 339-341.

4. What is Homeostasis. Scientific American. [Online] 2000. [Cited: November 8, 2019.] https://www.scientificamerican.com/article/what-is-homeostasis/.

5. International, QA. Visual Dictionary. QA International. [Online] 2019. [Cited: November 8, 2019.] http://www.ikonet.com/en/visualdictionary/static/us/hormones.

6. Effects of estrone, estradiol, and estriol on hormone-responsive human breast cancer in long-term tissue culture. Lippman, M., Monaco, M.E., & Bolan G. 6, 1977, Cancer Research, Vol. 37, pp. 1901-1907.

7. Estrogen hormone biology. Hamilton, K.J., Hewitt, S.C., Arao, Y., & Korach, K. s.l. : Current Topics in Developmental Biology, 2017, Vol. 125, pp. 109-146.

8. Estradiol: A hormone with diverse and contradictory neuroprotective actions. . Wise, P.M., Suzuki, S., & Brown, C.M. 3, 2009, Translational Research, Vol. 11, pp. 297-303.

9. Obesity and breast cancer: The estrogen connection. Cleary, M.P., Grossman, M.E. 6, 2009, Endocrinology, Vol. 150, pp. 2537-2542.

10. The natural history of the metabolic syndrome in young women with the polycystic ovary syndrome and the effect of long-term oestrogen-progestagen treatment. Pasquali, R., Gambineri, A., Anconetani, B.,. 1999, Clinical Endocrinology, Vol. 50, pp. 517-527. Clin Endocrinol (Oxf) . 1999;50:517–527..

11. Carmina, E., Campagna, A.M., Lobo, R.A. 2012, Obstetrics and Gynecology, Vol. 119, pp. 263-269. . 2012;119:263–269..

12. Determinants of menarche. Karapanou, O., Papadimitrou, A. 2010, Reproductive Biology and Endocrinology, Vol. 8, p. 115.

13. Has age at menarche changed? Results from the National Health and Nutrition Examination Survey (NHANES) 1999-2004. McDowell, M.A., Brody, D.J., Hughes, J.P. 3, 2007, Journal of Adolescent Health, Vol. 40, pp. 227-231.

14. Association of phthalates, parabens and phenols found in personal care products with pubertal timing in girls and boys. Harley, K.G., Berger, K.P., Kogut, K., Parra, K., Lustig, R.H., Greenspan, L.C., ... Eskenazi, B. 1, 2019, Vol. 34, pp. 109-117.

15. Perimenopausal and postmenopausal health. Cheung, A.M., Chaudhry, R., Kapral, M., Jackevicius, C., Robinson, G. 2004, BMC Womens Health, Vol. 4, p. S23.

16. Differences in age at death according to smoking and age at menopause. Bellavia, A., Wolk, A., Orsini, N. 2016, Menopause, Vol. 23, pp. 108-110.

17. 11 Harmful Effects of Smoking on Women's Health. [Online] n.d. Women.Smokefree.gov..

18. Effect of REM sleep deprivation on the antioxidant status in the brain of Wistar rats. Mathangi, D.C., Shyamala, R., Subhashini, A.S. 4, 2012, Annals of Neuroscience, Vol. 19, pp. 161-164.

19. Sleep and metabolism: An overview. Sharma, S., Kavuru, M. 2010, International Journal of Endocrinology, Vol. 270832.

20. Mitchell, G. The importance of self-care. Australian Menopause Center. [Online] 2019. [Cited: November 10, 2019.] https://www.menopausecentre.com.au/information-centre/articles/the-importance-of-self-care/.

21. Association of hormonal contraception with depression. Skovlund, C.W., Morch, L.S., Kessing, L.V., Lidegaard, O. 11, 2016, JAMA, Vol. 73, pp. 1154-1162.

22. Pharmacology of estrogens and progestogens: Influences of different routes of administration. Kuhl, H. 2005, Climacteric, Vol. 8, pp. 3-63.

23. Guttmacher Institute. Contraceptive Use in the United States. [Online] July 2018. [Cited: November 9, 2019.] https://www.guttmacher.org/fact-sheet/contraceptive-use-united-states.

24. Ovarian reserve assessment in users of oral contraception seeking fertility advice on their reproductive system. Birch Peterson, K., Hvidman, H.W., Forman, J.L., Pinborg, A., Larsen, E.C., ... & Andersen, A.N. 10, 2015, Human Reproduction, Vol. 30, pp. 2364-2375.

25. Hatcher, R.A., Nelson, A.L., Trussell, J., Cwiak, C., Cason, P., Policar, M.S., ... & Kowal, D. Contraceptive Technology. 21st ed. New York : Ayer Company Publishers, Inc., 2018.

26. Risk assessment of using aluminum foil in food preparation. . Bassioni, G., Mohammed, F.S., Zubaidy, E.A., Kobrsi, I. 7, 2012, International Journal of Electrochemistry., pp. 4498-4509.

27. Therapy of climacteric complaints with cimicifuga racemosa: Herbal medicine with clinically proven evidence. . Liske, E., Wustenbery, P. 1998, Menopause, Vol. 5, p. 350.

28. Suspected black cohosh hepatotoxicity. Naser, B., Schnitker, J., Minkin, M.J., De Arriba, S.G., Nolte, K.L., Osmers, R. 4, 2011, Menopause, Vol. 18, pp. 366-375.

29. Spontaneous reports of assumed herbal hepatotoxicity by black cohosh: Is the liver-unspecific Naranjo scale precise enought to ascertain causality?

Teschke, R., Schmidt-Taenzer, W., Wolff, A. 6, 2011, Pharmacoepidemiology and Drug Safety, Vol. 20, pp. 567-582.

30. Beneficial effects of Lepidium meyenii (Maca) on psychological symptoms and measures of sexual dysfunction in postmenopausal women are not related to estrogen or androgen content. Brooks, N.A., Wilcox, G., Walker, K.Z., Ashton, J.F., Cox, M.B., Stojanovska, L. 6, 2008, Menopause, Vol. 15, pp. 1157-1162.

31. The effect of vitamin D on hot flashes in menopausal women. Ziaei, S., Kazemnejad, A., Zareai, M. 4, 2007, Gynceology and Obstetric Investigation, Vol. 64, pp. 204-207.

32. High glycemic index diet as a risk factor for depression: Analyses from the Women's Health Initiative. Gangwisch, J.E., Hale, L., Garcia, L., Malaspina, D., Opler, M.G., Payne, M.E., Rossom, R.C., Lane, D. 2, 2015, American Journal of Clinical Nutrition, Vol. 102, pp. 454-463.

33. Harvard Health Publishing, Harvard Medical School. Don't give up on losing weight and staying fit. Harvard Women's Health Watch. [Online] August 2013. [Cited: November 15, 2019.] https://www.health.harvard.edu/staying-healthy/dont-give-up-on-losing-weight-and-staying-fit.

34. Select Committee on Nutrition and Human Needs. Dietary Goals for the United States. Washington DC : U.S. Government Printing Office, 1977.

35. Increased consumption of refined carbohydrates and the epidemic of type 2 diabetes in the United States: an ecologic assessment. Gross, L.S., Li, L., Ford, E.S., Liu, S. 5, 2004, American Journal of Clinical Nutrition, Vol. 79, pp. 774-779.

36. The effects of a low-carbohydrate, ketogenic diet on the polycystic ovary syndrome: A pilot study. Mavropoulos, J.C., Yancy, W.S., Hepburn, J., Westman, E.C. 2005, Nutrition and Metabolism, Vol. 2, p. 35.

37. Cholesterol in food. Heart Foundation. [Online] [Cited: November 15, 2019.] https://www.heartfoundation.org.au/healthy-eating/food-and-nutrition/fats-and-cholesterol/cholesterol-in-food.

38. MarketData. The U.S. Weight Loss & Diet Control Market. [Online] February 2019. [Cited: December 27, 2019.] https://www.marketresearch.com/Marketdata-Enterprises-Inc-v416/Weight-Loss-Diet-Control-12225125/?progid=91444.

39. Capsaicin and capsiate could be appropriate agents for treatment of obesity: A meta-analysis of human studies. Zsiboras, C., Matics, R., Hegyi, P., Balasko, M., Petervari, E., Szabo, I., ... Solymar, M. 9, Critical Reviews in Food Science and Nutrition, Vol. 58, pp. 1419-1427.

40. Green tea extract ingestion, fat oxidation, and glucose tolerance in healthy humans. Venables, M.C., Hulston, C.J., Cox, H.R., Jeukendrup, A.E. 3, 2008, American Journal of Clinical Nutrition., Vol. 87, pp. 778-784.

41. Effect of green tea or green tea extract consumption on body weight and body composition: Systematic review and meta-analysis. Baladia, E., Basulto, J., Manera, M., Martinez, R., Calbet, D. 3, 2014, Nutricion Hospitalaria, Vol. 29, pp. 479-490.

42. Midlife activity predicts risk of dementia in older male twin pairs. Carlson, M.C., Helms, M.J., Steffens, D.C., Burke, J.R., Potter, G.G., Plassman, B.L. 5, 2008, Alzheimer's & Dementia, Vol. 4, pp. 324-331.

43. Mindfulness-Based Stress Reduction in Post-treatment Breast Cancer Patients: Immediate and Sustained Effects Across Multiple Symptom Clusters. Reich, R.R., Lengacher, C.A., Alinat, C.B., Kip, K.E., Paterson, C., Ramesar, S., ... & Park, J.Y. 1, 2017, Journal of Pain and Symptom Management., Vol. 53, pp. 85-95.

44. Mindfulness practice leads to increases in regional brain gray matter density. Holzel, B.K., Carmody, J., Vangel, M., Congleton, C., Yerramsetti, S.M., Gard, T., Lazar, S.W. 1, 2011, Psychiatry Research, Vol. 191, pp. 36-43.

45. Long-chain omega-3 fatty acids and the brain: a review of the independent and shared effects of EPA, DPA and DHA. Dyall, S.C. 2015, Frontiers in Aging Neuroscience., Vol. 7, p. 52.

46. A double-blind, placebo-controlled, randomized trial of Ginkgo biloba extract EGb 761 in a sample of cognitively intact older adults: neuropsychological findings. Mix, J.A., Crews, W.D. Jr. 6, 2002, Human Psychopharmacology, Vol. 17, pp. 267-277.

47. Cognitive performance, SPECT, and blood viscosity in elderly non-demented people using Ginkgo biloba. Santos, R.F., Galduroz, J.C., Barbieri, A., Castiglioni, M.L., Ytaya, L.Y., Bueno, O.F. 4, 2003, Pharmachopsychiatry, Vol. 36, pp. 127-133.

48. Soybean-derived phosphatidylserine improves memory function of the elderly Japanese subjects with memory complaints. . Kato-Kataoka, A., Sakai, M., Ebina, R., Nonaka, C., Asano, T., Miyamori, T. 3, 2010, Journal of Clinical Biochemistry and Nutrition, Vol. 47, pp. 246-255.

49. Effects of resveratrol on memory performance, hippocampal functional connectivity, and glucose metabolism in healthy older adults. Witte, A.V., Kerti, L., Margulies, D.S., Floel, A. 23, 2014, The Journal of Neuroscience, Vol. 34, pp. 7862-7870.

50. Foods, fortificants, and supplements: Where do Americans get their nutrients? Fulgoni, V.L., Keast, D.R., Bailey, R.L., Dwyer, J. 2011, Journal of Nutrition., Vol. 141, pp. 1847-1854.

51. Aging and Sleep. National Sleep Foundation. [Online] December 2009. [Cited: November 17, 2019.] https://www.sleepfoundation.org/articles/aging-and-sleep.

52. Circadian clock function is disrupted by environmental tobacco/cigarette smoke, leading to lung inflammation and injury via a SIRT1-BMAL1 pathway. Hwang, J.W., Sundar, I.K., Yao, H., Sellix, M.T.,

Rahman, R. 1, 2014, The Federation of American Societies for Experimental Biology Journal, Vol. 28.

53. Higher prevalence of smoking in patients diagnosed as having obstructive sleep apnea. . Kashyap, R., Hock, L.M., Bowman, T.J. 4, 2001, Sleep and Breathing, Vol. 5, pp. 167-172.

54. Cortisol as a marker for improvment in mindfulness-based stress reduction. Matousek, R.H., Dobkin, P.L., Pruessner, J. 2010, Complementary therapies in clinical practice, Vol. 16, pp. 13-19.

55. The effects of mindfulness-based stress reduction on objective and subjective sleep parameters in women with breast cancer: a randomized controlled trial. Lengacher, C.A., Reich, R.R., Paterson, C.L., Jim, H.S., Ramesar, S., Alinat, C.B., ... & Kip, K.E. 4, 2015, Psychooncology, Vol. 24, pp. 424-432.

56. Cannabidiol in anxiety and sleep: A large case series. Shannon, S., Lewis, N., Lee, H., Hughes, S. 2019, The Permanente Journal, Vol. 23, pp. 18-41.

57. Hypnotic and antiepileptic effects of cannabidiol. Carlini, E.A., Cunha, J.M. S1, 1981, Journal of Clinical Pharmacology, Vol. 21, pp. 417S-427S.

58. Silexan, an orally administered Lavandula oil preparation, is effective in the treatment of 'subsyndromal' anxiety disorder: a randomized, double-blind, placebo controlled trial. . Kasper, S., Gastpar, M., Muller, W.E., Volz, H.P., Moller, H.J., Dienel A., Schlafke, S. 5, 2010, International Clinical Psychopharmacology, Vol. 25, pp. 277-287.

59. Effects of L-theanine administration on stress-related symptoms and cognitive functions in health adults: A randomized controlled trial. Hidese, S., Ogawa, S., Ota, M., Ishida, I., Yasukawa, Z., Ozeki, M., Kunugi, H. 10, 2019, Nutrients, Vol. 11, p. E2362.

60. Valerian for sleep: A systematic review and meta-analysis. Bent, S., Padula, A., Moore, D., Patterson, M., Mehling, W. 12, 2006, American Journal of Medicine, Vol. 119, pp. 1005-1012.

61. Effect of 1-year, low-dose DHEA therapy on climacteric symptoms and female sexuality. Genazzani, A.R., Stomati, M., Valentino, V., Pluchino, N., Pot, E., Casarosa, E., ... Luisi, M. 6, 2011, Vol. 14, pp. 661-668. .

62. Maca: An Andean crop with multi-pharmacological functions. Wang, Y., Wang, Y., McNeil, B., Harvey, L.M. 7, 2007, Food Research International, Vol. 40, pp. 783-792.

63. Effect of spearmint (Mentha spicata Labiatae) teas on androgen levels in women with hirsutism. Akdogan, M., Tamer, M.N., Cure, E., Cure, M.C., Koroglu, B.K., Delibas, N. 5, 2007, Phytotherapy Research , Vol. 21, pp. 444-447.

64. Spearmint herbal tea has significant anti-androgen effects in polycystic ovarian syndrome. A randomized controlled trial. Grant, P. 2, 2010, Phytotherapy Research, Vol. 24, pp. 186-188.

65. Effects of Zinc Supplementation on Endocrine Outcomes in Women with Polycystic Ovary Syndrome: a Randomized, Double-Blind, Placebo-Controlled Trial. Jamilian, M., Foroozanfard, F., Bahmani, F., Talaee, R., Monavari, M., Asemi, Z. 2, 2016, Biological Trace Element Research, Vol. 170, pp. 271-278.

66. Diet and hair loss: Effects of nutrient deficiency and supplement use. Guo, E.L., Katta, R. 1, 2017, Dermatology Practical & Conceptual, Vol. 7, pp. 1-10.

67. Watch, Harvard Women's Health. What's the scoop on bone soup? Harvard Health Publishing. [Online] 2015. [Cited: December 24, 2019.] https://www.health.harvard.edu/healthy-eating/whats-the-scoop-on-bone-soup.

68. Importance of estrogen receptors in adipose tissue function. Bluher, M. 3, 2013, Molecular Metabolism, Vol. 2, pp. 130-132.

69. Xenoestrogen exposure and mechanisms of endocrine disruption. Singleton, D.W., & Khan, S.A. 8, 2003, Frontiers of Bioscience, Vol. 1, pp. s110-118.

70. Estrogen: The necessary evil for human health, and ways to tame it. Patel, S., Homaei, A., Raju, A.B., Meher, B.R. 2018, Biomedical Pharmacotherapy, Vol. 102, pp. 403-411.

71. Clinical review 97: Potential health benefits of dietary phytoestrogens: a review of the clinical, epidemiological, and mechanistic evidence. Tham, D.M., Gardner, C.D., Haskell, W.L. 83, 1998, Journal of Clinical Endocrinology & Metabolism, pp. 2223-2235.

ABOUT THE AUTHOR

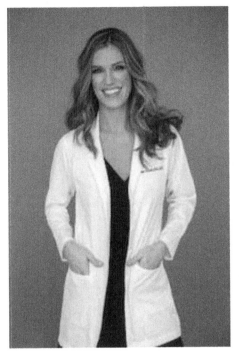

Dr. Carissa Alinat is an expert in weight loss and hormone balancing. She is also the author of a popular weight loss program, The French Paleo Burn.

She owns a busy clinic in Florida and has helped thousands of patients (especially women on menopause) reach their wellness goals and balance their hormones naturally.

Dr. Carissa's mission is to help women disrupt aging and live their best life past midlife.

Dr. Carissa obtained her PhD from the University of South Florida, where she has had extensive research experience in Complementary and Alternative Medicine while working on large clinical trials involving the use of Mindfulness-Based Stress Reduction in breast cancer survivors.

She has published more than 30 articles in medical journals and health magazines and has presented at conferences across the United States. She is also a board-certified nurse practitioner practicing in weight management and hormone therapy.
But first and foremost, she is a woman. She knows what it's like to feel tired all the time while riding on a hormonal rollercoaster and trying to keep it together. She has struggled with her own weight and hormone imbalances. She tried countless diets, took the wrong supplements, and failed over and over again until she finally found the solutions that helped her succeed.

She lives in Florida with her chef husband and their 5 children. They often travel to their second home in the South of France.

For more information on Dr. Carissa, to connect with her on social media, or for media inquiries, please visit her website at DoctorCarissa.com.

Made in the USA
Columbia, SC
17 August 2020